5 STEPS

TO BEING YOUR OWN
PATIENT
ADVOCATE

5 STEPS

TO BEING YOUR OWN
PATIENT ADVOCATE

STEPS

MY HEALTH. MY BODY. MY VOICE.
DR. CRISTY KESSLER

—— WITH SHARON MILLER ——

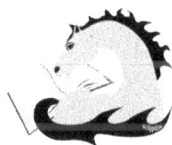

Buckskin Books
Tucson, Arizona

Coming in 2014
www.5stepsadvocate.com
See page 171

To Liz

We chose the road less traveled, walked it to the beat of our own drummer, laughed until we cried, and still have enough faith and love to last a lifetime.

To Jim

You have always been there with me and for me. Thank you for your love and support.

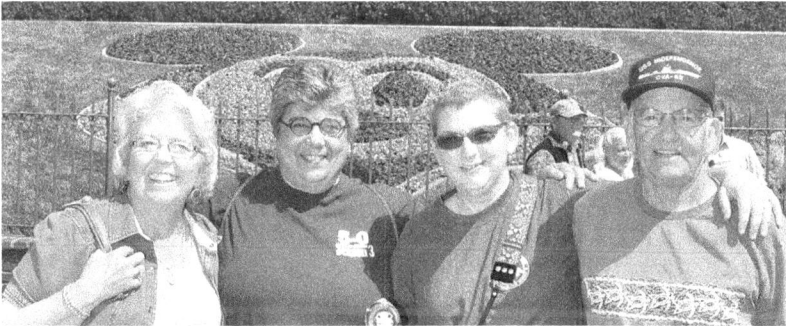

Sharon, Liz, Cristy, and Jim in Disneyland, 2013, celebrating life, love, happiness, and a bright future.

Modern medicine, for all its advances, knows less than ten percent of what your body knows instinctively.
—Deepak Chopra

Contents

ACKNOWLEDGMENTS

First and foremost I would like to thank Liz and Sharon. This book would not be possible without their love for me. Thank you, Liz, for giving me the space to get my story on paper and loving me enough to let me be. Jim and Jeff, thank you for letting me borrow your wife and mother. Her love for you is immeasurable.

Don, I finally finished the book we always talked about. I miss you every day.

Uncle Fuzzy, Cousin Phoebe, Uncle Butch, although you are not with me, you're with me in every word on every page.

My family: The Kesslers, The Buchanans, The Joneses, The Extended Zivanovs, The Millers, The Petrosinos, and the Patemans

Brandon, Edwin, Kristal, Lauren, Adriana, Javier, Reagan, Dylan, Thomas, Makena, Deniz: You are the future and I walked this journey in hopes you never have to. But if you do, just take it one step at a time.

Janet Kwan, cyberspace connected us, and you put in motion everything I needed to be alive today.

The Turkey Team: Dr. Gülbaş, you really are a gift from God. Dilek Inci, we met as patient/advocate and now we are family. Banu and your nursing staff—I forgive you for the daily 6 a.m. wake up and hypodermic needles. Meral, I appreciate all of the work you did on my behalf while I was at Anadolu.

Everyone at Anadolu Medical Center including all the other doctors, nurses, administrative staff, and support staff whose names I've forgotten. Anadolu Titanic Comfort Hotel, our home away from home with the best staff in the world.

The Hawaii Team: Dr. Uramoto, you believed when no one else would. You are a superstar quarterback! Lory, you are as important to my health care journey as any doctor. Past, current, and future players on my defensive line, your protected me when I needed it.

The One of Our Own Team, who really made things happen. Dave and Jill Randall for always making sure my story was heard and believing I was worth saving.

Nancy, you put together an amazing fundraiser in Maryland. Your energy and creativity made it a memorable night. And Richard, at Buontempo's, thanks for hosting the shindig at the best little Italian restaurant in Maryland.

Each and every donor: Whether you gave a little or a lot, every penny made a HUGE difference. God bless you all.

The Parish of St. Clement, University of Hawaii at Manoa College of Education, Rev Michael, Jiro, Amanda Doty, Bishop Bob Fitzpatrick, Suzie, Dan Leonard, Debbie Grisham, Jimmy Buffett's at the Beachcomber, Dr. Kimo Cashman, and the Sisters of St. Margaret in Boston.

Jenne, Sonya, Abby, Lisa for touching bases with me every day during the transplant, making me laugh with your cards, and feeding my sugar addiction.

My students from Perryville High School, my basketball players, Kenton for keeping me passionate about things that matter.

Michael Seres, from the moment we exchanged tweets I knew you were a special angel. You inspired me to put pen to paper.

Michelle Sismar for your friendship and keeping my hair as close to bald as possible

The MasterChef Season 2 crew, recovery was just so much easier. Ben, Adrien, Christian, Tracy, Jennifer you carry forth my mission of paying it forward. We ARE 'Ohana. Chef Graham Elliot, you matter.

Sidney Kessler, Thomas Cranmer Zivanov, Richard Hooker Zivanov, Bailey Kessler, Bristol Kessler, Leah Kessler, Nicholas Ridley Zivanov, St. Alban, Sir Dibley, St. Augustine, Cambridge, Kekoa McElroy, Hannah Miller.

Special thanks to those readers and reviewers who helped us make this book work: Linda "Lucy" Fernandez, Ben Starr, Dr. Tracie Umaki, Beth Pateman, Rev. Dr. Dennis Maynard, Lisa Thelen, Maya Soetoro-Ng.

And to our tireless proofreaders, Kim McKay Campbell and John Kennedy, THANKS!

FOREWORD

I first met Cristy Kessler on social media when we discovered that we had both been through a transplant. My own was as an intestinal transplant, the result of living with the long-term chronic condition Crohn's Disease and then intestinal failure. Cristy's was a whole different matter. We became great friends and I began to learn and understand the struggle that resulted in her stem cell transplant.

What became obvious straight away was that despite her own adversity, all she was really interested in was helping others. I learnt that, having become an associate professor and teacher at the University of Hawaii, her passion was to share her experiences and use them to make her a better communicator and person.

Like Cristy's, my own journey has been a long and often arduous one. My transplant was a result of over twenty surgeries, and in the build up to it I turned to social media and more specifically a blog to share my story. My journey into social media led me to understand further the power of patient-to-patient interactions as part of a healthcare journey. The ability to talk to someone who had experienced problems similar to yours, to share hints and tips, and to be a trusted source was invaluable. What I also learnt was that, like Cristy, the more you cope with your illness the more you become an expert in it. You end up understanding more about your condition than many professionals, and that can be a very valuable tool.

I have been fortunate enough to have had a clinical team open minded enough and brave enough to allow me to engage with them in ways never previously seen in healthcare. I have been able to use digital technologies to help navigate my way through the system and ultimately improve my healthcare outcomes. In an age of self-management, of remote monitoring, and of the patient taking on more responsibility, I was able to live that journey and hopefully share my experiences to help others.

Patients with long-term chronic conditions are becoming the biggest financial burden on healthcare. However, as more people are diagnosed with these conditions, knowing how to find a pathway through everything that comes their way is extremely hard. Cristy is uniquely positioned to help patients find their way through that maze. We have often talked at length about wanting to be part of every decision made about ours health care, and Cristy is living proof of a patient who has just done that. She successfully researched where the best treatments were and what the right medications should be. When she was told that she had to decamp half way around the world to receive the treatment, she simply did it.

With her book, she has been able to articulate in a very simple way the critical steps that every patient living with a long-term condition should abide by. She writes with complete honesty and lovely touches of humour. I remember meeting her for the first time in London and spending dinner either open mouthed in amazement at her courage or in fits of laughter at the stories she shared over the hospital she pretty much lived in whilst undergoing her own transplant. In many ways her book is not only a practical guide, but also an autobiographical account of large parts of her life.

So many of our lives are defined by our health: the decisions we make, the impact on our families, and the financial stresses that living with chronic illness causes. The fourth step in the book talks about Perseverance and Patience. From my own experience I would say that coping is as much a mental as physical challenge. Cristy understands that better than most. There were times when as patients it seems easier to lie down and cry. Cristy refers very articulately to the phrase most patients hate and that is "be patient." Well, I can tell you, too, it is very hard to stay patient and remain focused on the outcome. Her book is one of those that you will read from cover to cover but then often go back to for top ups and reminders of what to do when times are tough.

This book matters more than you will realise. No foreword can do real justice to the book; you simply have to read it. When Cristy talks about being "the coach of her team," you hear and feel her passion shining through. Underneath it all, though, she is right. If you are going to navigate your way through incredibly choppy waters (and let's face it, we all do at different times) then you have to learn to be the captain of your ship. The coach of your team.

Above all, I would say that this is a book every single patient should read at least once. And, if you are a clinician, then this should be on your bookshelf or on your laptop as a constant reminder of the paths and decisions we patients have to take. Don't get me wrong, it is hard being a long-term patient, but Cristy makes it a whole lot easier with her words. Sometimes, in our own little world of chronic illness, we think, no one can know what it feels like to say goodbye to your loved ones before a procedure and not know if you will ever see them again. Wrong, Michael— other patients do. Cristy didn't know if she would pull through. Somehow, through all that adversity, she came through it to share her experiences in such a way that it should become the go-to book for all patients' wishing to be their own advocates.

I am incredibly proud to call Cristy a friend and I am incredibly proud of this book. I hope you enjoy it and learn from it in the same way as I have.

Michael Seres, London, England
Michael's Website: www.michaelseres.com
Twitter: @mjseres
Michael's Blog, *Being a Patient Isn't Easy*:
http://beingapatient.blogspot.com

INTRODUCTION

If you do a Google search for the term "patient advocate" you get over 14,000,000 hits in about thirty seconds. It can be overwhelming; how do you find one advocate among millions who can help you navigate your medical journey? Or how do you use what you find to help others locate professionally trained advocates who will stand up for their best interests? Merriam-Webster defines an advocate as "one who pleads the cause for another or promotes and supports the interests of another." Exploring those links often provides a great deal of information about the work of a patient advocate. Most sites describe tangible, concrete tasks the advocate should perform in order to ensure their client (you or your loved one) is getting the best care in the hospital.

Advocates often provide us with lists of questions to ask before, during, and after diagnosis and treatment, tips for effective care giving once the client (again, you or your loved one) returns from the hospital, and even advice for caregiver needs. This guidance is priceless and, in many cases, serves as our field manual when we are faced with difficult healthcare issues for ourselves or for those we love.

The concept of a formal patient advocate is a fairly new phenomenon. The patient advocate's job is to maintain the patients' rights by educating them, responding to complaints from the patient or from the patient's family, and resolving issues on behalf of the patient. That said, one of the primary duties of the patient advocate is to make certain the patient and the family understand the hospital's policy on patient rights. Additionally, the advocate is responsible for preventing complaints and for documenting complaints when prevention fails. At times the patient advocate acts as a mediator between the hospital's legal department and patients who have complaints. Overall, the patient advocate's role is to help create a positive environment for patients and their families at what might be a very difficult time.

Many hospitals, insurance companies, and health care facilities employ professional patient advocates, but their loyalties may not lie entirely on the side of the patient, since it's not the patient who signs their paycheck. Some independent patient advocates are available for hire for those who can afford an objective advocate not swayed by the profit margin of the facility or organization. But this book is about the most powerful and loyal patient advocate you'll find anywhere...yourself.

5 S.T.E.P.S. to Being Your Own Patient Advocate outlines for you the steps you can follow to navigate the medical system as you search for answers, diagnoses, and treatment:

- **Step 1: Sensibility**—Listen to your body and learn how to interpret what it has to tell you so you can share this information with your doctors.

- **Step 2: Teamwork**—Build a team of medical practitioners and a family and friends support network that communicates well and works together for the same goals.

- **Step 3: Education**—Learn everything you can about the symptoms, disorders, diseases that you may be facing as well as the treatments available; become an expert on you.

- **Step 4: Patience and Perseverance**—Don't expect things to happen quickly, but don't give up; know when to push for more timely information and treatment.

- **Step 5: Sustainability**—This is all about you and what you need to take care of and protect your body, mind, and spirit. It involves deep thought and reflection to determine what you need in your life that will help you keep going day after day after day.

At the end of each chapter, you will find a short section called "Just Remember," which offers a succinct list of the important things you will want to take away from that chapter, and another section called "S.T.E.P.S. in Action," through which you will get a much clearer picture of my personal medical journey. Because the central content of the book is not presented in chronological order, but focused on the steps you need to take to be your own patient advocate, you may be left wondering about some of the details of my story. This feature will provide that.

I've also provided an extensive medical glossary to help you deal with the frequent use of medical terms, procedures, and medications throughout the book. If you are reading the e-book, the first use of these terms links to glossary entry which will enable you to read about it and then use the return link to pick up reading where you left off. If you are reading the print version, you're stuck with the old-fashioned, flip to the back of the book strategy. In any case, then, you can turn to the glossary when you encounter one of these medical terms for more information.

My central purpose, though, is to help anyone, novice or pro, maneuver within the health care system effectively. These steps are not intended to be absolute, but rather organic and easily adapted to fit into the medical journey that you call your own.

So come along with me as I share my experiences and the strategies I have developed that helped see me through my journey from waiting to die to learning to live.

CHAPTER 1—A LIFETIME OF PAIN AND ILLNESS

My name is Dr. Cristy Kessler, and **I should be dead**. I'm serious. I should be dead. All my life I've been plagued by a series of rare, ultimately lethal autoimmune disorders, as well as multiple types of cancer. When I was nearly forty years old, the medical community basically threw in the towel and told me there was nothing they could do for me. It was only by becoming my own patient advocate that I reclaimed my life and will to live, discovered, researched, and underwent a controversial stem cell transplant procedure, and became healthy and pain free for the first time in my entire life.

I'm forty-two now and for the first twenty-four years of my life I had no idea that there was something wrong. I thought everyone lived with pain. Hell, I thought everyone who got up in the morning had a hard time moving. But how could I know anything different? I had always had this pain for as long as I can remember. My first conscious memory of the stiffness and pain I felt when I put weight on my legs was when I was in preschool. I remember sitting on the reading rug and listening to Mrs. Macky. We were all sitting "criss-cross-applesauce" and when story time was over and we were supposed to lie down to have our naps, when I tried to move, a burning pain shot straight up and down my spine. With a jolt I sat straight up and immediately got scolded for not lying down. None of the other kids seemed to be bothered by this pain, so I lay down, curled into a ball, and cried silently until I fell asleep.

Oh, and by the way, I'm not that kind of doctor. Although I've been sick all my life, instead of a medical degree, I managed to earn a doctorate in education. My educational journey is another story, but I am proud of my achievements in spite of the pain and illnesses that were my constant companions on that journey. So navigating the health care system has been a new journey for me.

You may (rightly) ask, what exactly qualifies me to give advice on being your own patient advocate? It is a question I have been asking myself for the past three years as this book muddled its way around in my mind. But once I put the details of my health care experiences on paper, I quickly saw that I have, indeed, developed enough experience, over time, to begin to categorize my experiences into steps that could prove helpful to others. The chart below depicts major medical milestones in my adult life. I've included major procedures, major treatments, and major hospital visits for exploratory testing to find diagnoses or second opinions.

From the time I was twenty-four years old (1995) until age forty (2011), I had nine major procedures, three major treatment plans (which involved lengthy out-patient administration at the hospital or training from specialists at the hospital), two visits to major health care centers where I spent a week meeting various doctors of different specialties and having further testing done: the first in Bangkok, Thailand, to see if I was a candidate for a stem cell transplant, and the other in the U.S. to confirm what my rheumatologist diagnosed in Hawaii. I had been to eleven different hospitals located in three different states and two in foreign countries. All of this in sixteen years.

From birth until age twenty-two (when I graduated from college with my bachelor's degree), I spent a lot of time being sick. My parents can tell you I was always sick. Every holiday, every major vacation, every event...I would get sick. I had pneumonia too many times to count, mononucleosis with several recurrences according to my doctor. I was an expert at tonsillitis, bronchitis, and ear infections. My gastrointestinal (GI) tract was never very good. Eat anything with a tomato base after 6 p.m. and chances were very high I would be throwing up before midnight. I was not able to keep breast milk down at birth or the most common forms of baby formula. No, I needed to have a prescription for a special formula. As my sister has always said, "If there is going to be a health complication or a weird medical diagnosis, it will be my sister." I wore braces for four years just to have my teeth go crooked again (which I discovered much later is a symptom of scleroderma; it happens when the jaw bone constricts); I had a severe case of dry sockets associated with my wisdom teeth being pulled out; during my hysterectomy I ended up with a hole in my bladder for which I had a catheter for three weeks while it healed. If it could happen as a potential risk or side effect to medication or a procedure, I would get it.

With all this being said, it is okay because through each experience I perfected my *5 S.T.E.P.S.* and I know they work, not just for the patient but also for the patient's team that patients choose to surround themselves with (loved ones, friends, family, and doctors).

Major Medical Events

Date	Location	
Treatment: Alternative Medication	1998–2003	University of Maryland Medical Center (MD)
Treatment: Methotrexate Injections (3 years)	2007–2010	Queens POB 3 (HI)
Major Procedure: Gall Bladder	1995	Harford Memorial (MD)
Major Procedure: Achilles Tendon Repair	1996	Union Memorial (MD)
Major Procedure: Achilles Tendon Repair	2002	Mercy Medical Center (MD)

Major Procedure: Uterine Cancer/Hysterectomy	2005	Kapiolani Hospital (HI)
Major Procedure: Meckel's Divderticula and Cancerous Growth Removed	2006	Queen's Medical Center (HI)
Exploratory/2nd Opinion: Diagnostics	2007	Mayo Clinic (AZ)
Treatment: Chemotherapy/Cytoxin and Rituxin (1 year, every 3 months)	2010	Kapiolani Hospital (HI)
Exploratory/2nd Opinion: Stem Cell Transplant Exploratory Option	2010	Bangkok, Thailand
Major Procedure: Autologous Stem Cell Transplant	2011	Anadolu Medical Center (Turkey)

Between 2009 and 2011, I was turned down by eight different studies/clinical trials being conducted in the U.S. that would have given me the same procedure as provided at Anadolu Medical Center.

And Now

When it is all added up, my life has been a medical mystery with a variety of diagnoses being handed down. In 2000, when I was diagnosed and underwent surgery for Chiari malformation, I started to feel better, and I really believed my medical issues would be over for a long time. What I didn't expect was the need to continue to navigate the health care system, identifying and changing team players regularly, learning how to be patient, but also persevering when I needed to, and sustaining my mind and spirit throughout this journey into the medical world, a journey that turned into the most amazing, and sometimes terrifying, roller coaster rides.

When I was faced with making the decision to have a stem cell transplant, I was empowered by the many guides transplant centers make available online. My partner, Liz, and I learned how to navigate each stage of the transplant; we learned what to expect with common side effects; we researched information about the accreditation the hospital and transplant center should have, along with the credentials of the doctor who would lead the transplant team; and we made sure we knew how to communicate with my insurance company and the billing department at the hospital (Step 3). All of this is incredibly important information to have, so the question became one of who would be the advocate to speak for me when the decision was made and the time came for the transplant.

The problem for us was twofold. One, my insurance company would not pay for my life-saving transplant nor would the Food and Drug Administration (FDA) permit a qualified doctor in the United States to perform my transplant. Apparently, stem cell transplants are considered experimental for autoimmune diseases. Even though two separate doctors—one in Hawaii where I live and one on the mainland—agreed that I was a perfect candidate for it, I would not be considered for the procedure anywhere in the United States. Not even if I had a bucketful of cash to pay for it myself. As a result, I had to explore options for having the procedure somewhere outside of the United States, settling finally on Anadolu Medical Center near Istanbul, Turkey. (More about that later.)

Two, I wanted to be my own patient advocate. Not to misunderstand, I needed my partner to advocate for me at various times, and I'm quite sure I wouldn't be alive without my two patient advocates from WorldMed Assist and Anadolu Medical Center. The key is knowing that everything they did was guided by my ability to advocate for myself prior to starting the transplant process and my success in putting a powerful team into place (Step 2). My team included not just medical experts, but family and friends who supported me throughout the process. Without any doubt, everyone on my team was fully aware of my wishes and needs.

When I conceived of using my experiences to write a book that goes far beyond the tangible, specific steps provided in a typical patient advocate guide, I realized that I had a great deal to offer. Based on my own experience, this book outlines five steps that will help you be your own best advocate.

What this book is not is the be-all and end-all of patient advocacy. It is not intended to be used as a singular resource, but one used in combination with anything and everything that can bring you one step closer to a healthy you. You will still need those who will help you; these include your professional patient advocates, your family support system, and all of those you meet in your journey to diagnosis and treatment. The important thing to remember is that an educated you is a healthier you. I don't want to be your patient advocate; I want you to do it yourself (or at least to know enough to make sure you are getting the care you need).

For the purpose of this guide, I define health in terms of body, mind, and spirit. For those of us who have been diagnosed with incurable, chronic, and/or terminal conditions, health is never again considered normal in the ordinary sense; our normal means managing our symptoms (both mental and physical) and maintaining a spirit that can soar so we can persevere. Healthy means finding the "right" answers that are "right" for you, finding your new normal.

Hospitals, doctors, insurance companies all recognize the importance of patient advocacy, so why shouldn't we (as patients) also value its importance? Some organizations truly have your best interests as their motivation. Others, while almost impossible to prove, hire patient advocates primarily to protect themselves. In these cases, the patient advocate only presents the medical angle that the health provider feels is in their best interest. For example, the patient advocate at one medical center guided me through multiple appointments, duplicating diagnostic tests that I had had within the three months prior to my arrival and for which I had brought test results. When, after three days of diagnostics I thought were redundant, and being curious, I asked why I had not been able to see a specialist at that point. The patient advocate—after a moment of stunned silence during which she digested the question—finally responded. "Here, we do all of the preliminary testing and diagnostics ourselves because we need to be sure that they are done correctly." I saw this as somewhat arrogant, but I also wondered about how much additional revenue such unnecessary testing provided for the clinic and to what degree the practice was designed, not for the patient, but for protecting the clinic.

To these providers a patient advocate is someone who can sit with you while you sign off on paperwork and "strongly encourage" you to follow company protocol. But what if you know (either intuitively or intellectually) you need something different? Something more? What if you need more information, a second or third opinion, or just need more processing time? Bottom line, what about you?

On March 21, 2011, I was given a new life. I was the recipient of an autologous stem cell transplant (SCT). Today, I AM ALIVE! My transplant and my story are unique. As I said before, I could not have my transplant done in the United States of America because the FDA had not approved SCT for my specific autoimmune diseases, and I did not fit nicely into an FDA-sanctioned research study—apparently, I wasn't "dead enough." Had I been closer to death I might have qualified, but I was told that even if I did qualify, the success rate was quite low. One has to wonder if the success rate was somehow the result of waiting too long to put patients into the program. Didn't anyone wonder if they would have more success by offering the treatment earlier? Apparently, patient advocacy was and is lacking for this research.

Facing disability from work and a slow death, I had two choices: Wait to die; or learn to live. I chose to live, which meant I needed to find someone in the world who believed that health care needs to be proactive, not reactive. With my faith and Internet determination, I found my answers.

CHAPTER 2—STEP 1: SENSIBILITY

Too much sensibility creates unhappiness and too much insensibility creates crime.
Charles de Talleyrand

The word, sensibility, should be easy enough to define, and as the first step in anyone's journey to becoming her own patient advocate makes a lot of sense—no pun intended. You cannot help but think about the many ways we use the word and its relatives: good sense, common sense, sixth sense, sensible, making sense (or not), five senses, come to one's senses, in a sense, nonsense, to sense something is wrong, sharpen one's senses. Most of us have heard of the book *Sense and Sensibility,* but how likely is it we understand the distinction Jane Austen tried to make between the two terms?

What does this term mean to me and why did I choose it as the first step in becoming your own patient advocate? What does it mean, really? Sometimes, I tell myself it means to be sensible. Clever to think I can still employ basic word building techniques I learned in elementary school. But it is really more than just being sensible; to really get to the "heart" of the word, I have to dig a little deeper and describe it in terms of how it looks and feels to me.

For me, it means knowing what I am feeling and how my body responds to whatever is happening to it. Merriam-Webster defines it in their medical dictionary as "the ability to receive sensations and the awareness of and responsiveness toward something." It is sometimes thought of as an acute perception of or responsiveness to something. You, then, as a patient facing life-threatening illness, must depend on your ability to perceive of and respond to the emotional and physical stimuli you encounter as you navigate the medical maze toward a diagnosis and treatment. How do you focus on navigating this maze when your body is wracked with pain or when debilitating symptoms distract you from your goal? Your acute perception of and response to the brutal stimuli that often accompany major illnesses may sometimes be as much as you can handle. How do you set aside those perceptions and responses in order to attend to those associated with your medical journey? It is often a heroic task, and even more so when you encounter the sometimes clinical indifference of health care workers and medical staff within the maze.

As I mentioned in the introduction, my own medical journey has been very long and involved. It has never been just one thing, but rather a constellation of experiences that have helped me perfect the craft of navigating the health care system, something that drives me to share my journey and my "road map" with you.

When you start life living in constant pain, it is hard to determine whether something different is a problem or if it is just part of your "normal." I'm being completely honest when I tell you that I really believed everyone felt the same pain and discomfort I did—it was, simply, my life. It came, then, as a huge shock to me that the pain I felt as my "normal" was, in fact, not everyone else's "normal," I began to understand this when I was in high school. It took breaking down in tears during soccer practice one afternoon in tenth grade to learn that my pain was not the norm.

In spite of the pain, or maybe because of it, I became a hell of an athlete as a youngster. I was Daddy's girl, a tomboy, intending to grow up to be a ball player—almost any ball would do. For my size, and in spite of how my body felt, I was fast, agile, and extremely determined. I was raised to believe that failure was not an option and to accept the

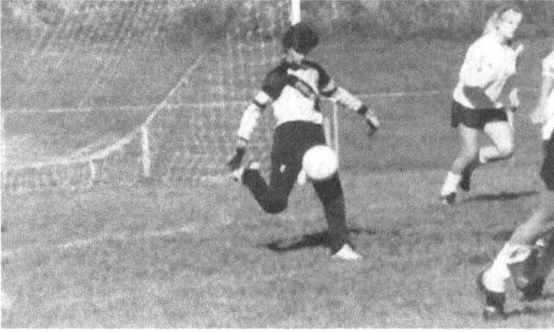
Cristy in the goal for C. Milton Wright High School

athletic adage, "No pain, no gain." Because of that, I was convinced that the pain I felt after any physical activity was normal for all people, all ages, all athletes. I had to prove myself. It started with baseball and softball, then basketball (playing in an all-boys' league) followed by soccer. I excelled in softball and even more so in soccer, earning All-State recognition in high school and a scholarship to a local community college (which started me on my educational journey), as well as earning national ranking as a college soccer goalie.

So there I was on a sunny afternoon on the soccer field at C. Milton Wright High School, in Maryland, in 1986. I was in the goal fielding practice shots from the left and right by my teammates. It was my favorite part of practice because I was involved in every shot. There was no standing around watching my teammates launch an assault on the opposing team's goal. There was no waiting for a ball to be kicked in my direction. It was challenging and almost always exhilarating.

About halfway through shooting practice, I suddenly broke down in tears. I left the goal box and went up to the hill to sit down. And I cried, I cried uncontrollably. I hurt. Every limb on my body was tingling and burning. I sat there crying and feeling like a total wimp. My coach was bewildered because this had never happened before. And nothing had happened during shooting practice that would have caused an injury; it had been a typical day like all the rest. Coach, who was and still is an amazing person and good friend, finally asked me what was going on. I told him my arms and legs were burning and tingling. He seemed embarrassed and perplexed, offering no answers or suggestions. (Years later, in November, 2011, at a fundraiser in Maryland for my medical expenses, Coach finally fessed up to thinking it was "just my time of month" and that I was overly emotional. We both enjoyed a great laugh since back then I wasn't sure what was wrong with me either.)

Finding My Way

After that breakdown, it occurred to me that none of my other friends or teammates had ever done anything even remotely similar, and I began to wonder whether they were just stronger than me or if, in fact, what was happening to me was somehow different. And so my quest began, albeit a little ineffectually at that time.

It was hard to make a commitment to this quest with school and family pressures that took precedence, but I always knew there was something I needed to know that I didn't have the resources for at the time. Making it through high school, earning the grade point average necessary to win a scholarship, attaining recognition for my athletic prowess, were all very important to me. These were the things I believed would somehow prove my value to the community, to the world. Winning acceptance in my family was to achieve great things. So my quest kept getting postponed and shoved aside in favor of these other goals.

Besides, information about these rather non-specific symptoms, which I later learned were indicative of autoimmune diseases, was not readily available. Those childhood illnesses—mono, strep infections, tonsillitis, pneumonia—cost me precious time at school and on the athletic fields. It also seemed to me that my inability to breast feed as an infant and to keep food down throughout childhood, might have been an indicator of something wrong. My mother, who is a registered nurse and a damned good one, might have suspected something if she had gotten her medical training sooner, but I was in school by the time she became an RN, and in those days—early 70s—

little was known about autoimmune diseases anyway. She would have tackled it with a vengeance if she had known.

Eventually, with symptoms becoming increasingly urgent and, in some cases, debilitating, along with multiple surgeries and procedures along the way, my quest to find out the "whys" for my pain led to the health care journey which I would ultimately endure over approximately sixteen years. It took me about six of those years to come to terms with the urgency of my health care and to develop a system that would garner the respect of the medical team which joined me on this journey.

I am not one who keeps a journal or feels comfortable with that process. In fact, I have a tendency to rebel against it because it had been shoved down my throat in graduate and postgraduate school. Journaling is not something you do because someone makes you do it; if you choose to journal, it comes from somewhere inside and it offers positive emotional rewards. I just didn't get it.

Frequently, hospital-employed patient advocates advised me to keep a daily journal of my feelings and symptoms. I wasn't motivated to follow their instructions when there weren't any guidelines for how to use such a journal with my doctors. Have you ever tried to give a doctor a journal that resembles a diary, and say, "Here, this will explain it all for you." I actually did that, and my efforts at journaling were largely ignored because a doctor's time is so limited. It's unreasonable to expect doctors to wade through your journal looking for clues to a diagnosis, and it's probably true that those patient advocates rarely collaborated with the doctors on the value of patient journaling.

As a result, I developed a system that would work more effectively, providing the conversation starter at each doctor's appointment. As I sit and put together this chapter, I can't even begin to tell you how much I wish someone had provided me with a plan like this. I believe it would have saved six years of frustrating doctor appointments. But before you throw up your arms and say, "Here we go, another 'expert' telling me what works," I encourage you to keep reading to see if any part of my example, no matter how small or large, could be used as a system of sensibility for your health care journey. I promise I am not dictating to you how to do this, but rather illustrating that it has helped me to be alive today.

The T-Chart Strategy

My T-Chart strategy developed by first throwing away my journal and pulling out a sheet of graph paper (although now I do it on the computer using a spreadsheet). I made a list of every symptom and issue I was experiencing. I did this quickly as a brainstorming activity, no more than three minutes. By limiting the time I had to make the list I found that the most important issues were the ones on my mind at that exact time and in that exact space. When my stopwatch beeped at the three-minute mark, I reviewed

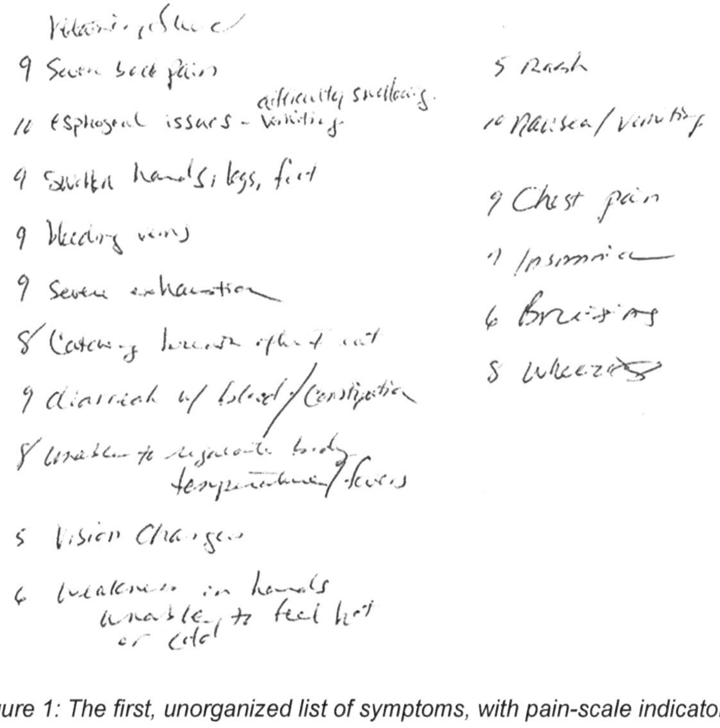

Figure 1: The first, unorganized list of symptoms, with pain-scale indicators.

my list and asked myself, out loud, if this was an honest set of symptoms. Being honest with yourself is key. I need to point out, though, that you might look at a symptom, like swollen hands, and think to yourself this is probably a minor issue for a doctor; however, you need to leave it on the list because it was one of stimuli that triggered your response—your sensibility. If it is important to you, then the doctor needs to value that importance and not dismiss the symptom as minor or irrelevant.

The next step is to review the list again and rate each one on a pain scale from 1 – 10 (See Figure 1). I used a standard pain scale, the Faces Pain Scale-Revised from the International Association for the Study of Pain. Assign an honest number based on the five days right before your doctor's appointment. A mistake I made early on was assigning higher pain numbers to my symptoms than was accurate in hopes my doctor would then be moved to

Dr. Y   9/10/10

Urgent   Secondary

Swallowing   Back pain
Vomiting   Swollen hands/feet/legs
bleeding veins   diarrhea with blood or constipation
exhaustion   No in between
catching breath after   Vision changes
     I eat   Weakness in hands can't feel
Fevers/normal body temp   hot or cold
     running low   rash
Chest pain → not   Insomnia
  heart, @ lungs   Bruising
unable to take   wheezing
deep breath w/o
pain around rib
cage

Figure 2: The symptom list, reorganized into the T-Chart

believe it. The interesting thing is when you find a doctor who does value your sensibility, the level of pain is less important than the fact you have a symptom at all.

After rating each symptom, the next thing is to divide the list into two categories—Urgent and Secondary—and place them on a new T-Chart, which is the one I take with me to the doctor (See Figures 2 and 3). It's easy to read and gives the doctor a quick summary of what has been happening to you. The first time I took my T-Chart into the office visit with me, I handed a copy to my doctor and kept one for myself. I explained to him what he was reading. His response was, "Holy cow. This is awesome." I told him that things in the Secondary category meant that they had been non-existent over the last five days because I had found ways to manage or control them and reduce their effect on my daily life. I also told him this list is always changing, and just because something had been non-existent in the previous five days, it didn't mean those symptoms wouldn't emerge as urgent later on. His response was, "Cool. This does give us a good place to start."

When I opened myself to the task of writing down my symptoms, not on a daily basis, mind you, but once a week,

September 10, 2010   Pain Management Specialist

URGENT	SECONDARY
Swallowing	Back pain
Vomiting	Swollen hands/feet/legs
Bleeding veins	Diarrhea with blood or constipation. Nothing in between
Exhaustion	Vision changes
Catching breath after I eat	Weakness in hands, can't feel hot or cold things
Fevers/normal body temp running low	Rash
Chest pain, not my heart, area around lungs unable to take deep breaths w/o pain around rib cage	Insomnia
	Bruising easily
	Wheezing

Figure 3: A neater copy for the doctor, but only if you feel up to it. Handwritten is good, too.

it changed my relationship with my doctors. Historically, I was the patient who, when the doctor asked, "What seems to be the issue?" I would start talking and they would interrupt to ask a question, and I would inevitably forget my thought or end up going off on a tangent. My T-Chart served as a conversation starter and a way for me to track changes over time, as well as maintaining a record of constant, persistent symptoms that were not changing no matter what medical protocol was used.

So What?

By now you may be asking, "What makes this any different from the practical advice you find from professional patient advocates or other sources?" The answer is nothing, in terms of preparing for your doctor appointments with a tangible list of concrete details to share. But the answer is everything, in terms of your mind and spirit. It is essential for maintaining an awareness of your sensibilities (STEP 1), and it establishes the foundation for the remaining four steps toward being your own patient advocate.

Developing your sensibilities regarding what you feel and how you respond to the symptoms you experience will not be of much value unless you can communicate clearly and completely with your medical team. You are:

- laying the groundwork for a communication bridge with your medical team, of which you are an important member **(STEP 2)**;

- educating yourself about your health issues, and, in fact, becoming an expert in the field of you, which goes far beyond simply doing the research and reading about your medical problems **(STEP 3)**;

- balancing perseverance with patience, that is, giving your medical team time to do what they need to do, but recognizing when you need to give someone a push in order to make something happen in the sometimes crazy world of medical care **(STEP 4)**;

- hanging tough, staying the course, and sustaining the effort until you find relief from your illness **(STEP 5)**.

No one knows your body like you do. Not even the best of the best doctors can fully understand you as well as you do.

My Story

Before I had perfected my approach to medical care, I spent a great deal of time trying to look inward to find the source of my pain and the symptoms I was experiencing. For some reason, I believed I could find the answers within myself, that somehow, someday, my body would surrender to my demands and give me the answers. I wanted to know why my entire body was swollen up, why I was gaining weight in spite of a decreased appetite (sometimes gaining two pounds in a weekend), why I would experience slurred speech, vertigo, and hives on the palms of my hands, and why, if I sneezed, I would have a major migraine headache for two to three days.

In hindsight, I know now that all of these symptoms are directly linked to autoimmune disease, but because I didn't have a positive ANA test (which detects antinuclear antibodies in the blood, those evil antibodies that attack your own body's cells, which is a clear indication of autoimmune disorders) or thickening of the skin, autoimmune disease was dismissed.

As a matter of fact, it was around 1996, when I was twenty-five years old, that my GP, whom I had been with for five years, dismissed my symptoms, telling me they were "all in my head." Frustrated and belittled, I left his office feeling as if I was, in fact, crazy. Even after doing blood work, x-rays, and referring me to rheumatology at Johns Hopkins Hospital in Baltimore, he told me that I was fine, physically, and that I needed to consider seeing a therapist to help me deal with my hypochondria. What he didn't know, or failed to remember (shouldn't the doctor read your chart?), was that I had been going to counseling for two years.

Indeed, it was my psychologist who was urging me to "stay the course," to find answers about my poor physical health. Because of the dejected feeling I got from my general practitioner and the sensibility of my counselor, I developed my T-Chart system. One week later, I returned to see my GP, T-Chart in hand, determined to be heard. The first sentence out of my mouth was, "Let's be sensible here. I'm educated, hardworking, and I know my body better than anyone. It is unacceptable to tell me everything I feel is all in my head." He stared at me and said nothing. I mean n-o-t-h-i-n-g. I pulled out my T-Chart and he actually sat down and read his copy. But don't even imagine that he experienced an epiphany and made a commitment to seeing me through treatment. In fact, I would only see him one more time.

Two years later, I called and made an appointment with him. I was on a mission to inform him he was, indeed, correct. My major health issue at the time was "all in my head." I had just had a Chiari malformation repair on my brain stem, which was the result of finding doctors who would listen to me and order the proper tests to identify the problem. I took a great deal of pleasure in telling him that I would never return to his office for any reason, but I wanted him to know, by showing him the MRIs of my brain stem, that I did have a major health issue, and when it was properly diagnosed and treated, it magically fixed everything that was wrong with my head. Too bad we didn't have cell phones with cameras back then. I would have his facial expression framed and hanging on my living room wall.

Summary

In the eighteenth century, sensibility was associated with the idea that through our senses, knowledge is gathered and, for some, it was considered a virtue. But then, according to Wikipedia, it became associated with *... an English-language literary movement, particularly in the then-new genre of the novel. Such works, called sentimental novels, featured individuals who were prone to sensibility, often weeping, fainting, feeling weak, or having fits in reaction to an emotionally moving experience... (http://en.wikipedia.org/wiki/Sensibility)*

Eventually, behaviors characterized as sensibilities were rejected as mere histrionics which had little to do with intellectual response or the attainment of any knowledge. This resulted in creating negative connotations for the notion of sensibility. Jane Austen's *Sense and Sensibility* was considered a "witty satire on the sentimental novel" because of her juxtaposition of the concepts of sense and reason with sensibility and feeling.

I prefer to believe that sense and reason and sensibility and feeling are not incompatible notions. For me, sensibility is a way of gathering knowledge. We can take advantage of our sensibilities, our reactions to physical and emotional stimuli, to build knowledge about the medical problems and needs of our bodies. Had I listened to the doctor who tried to convince me that my symptoms were not important, not related...or worse, not even real...I would be dead today.

As I said before, you are the expert on you. You are the only one who knows what is happening to your body, but the key lies in developing the skills to share those things rationally and sensibly to your doctors. This is especially true when you have a doctor like my GP who apparently saw me as a character in an eighteenth-century novel, prone to weeping, fainting, and hysteria.

The T-Chart I described here is an effective way to translate your sensibilities into sensible descriptions that will help your doctors recognize and understand your symptoms and join you on your journey to diagnosis and treatment.

Just Remember

- Pay attention to what your body is telling you.

- Make lists of symptoms and scale them using a reputable medical pain scale.

- Organize your list according to what is urgent and what is secondary.

- Take your list with you to the doctor so that nothing is overlooked in consultation.

- Don't let anyone, even a doctor, dismiss your symptoms.

- Prepare to take charge of your medical care.

You can download your own personal T-Chart Worksheet by visiting the 5 STEPS website at:

www.5stepsadvocate.com/download-t-chart.html

S.T.E.P.S. in Action: Sensibility

I spent my lifetime, it seems, being acutely aware of every feeling or stimulus in my body that may be a sign or symptom of illness. These days, I sometimes find myself feeling as if I've forgotten to do something important, and then I realize it was to make a T-Chart for the week.

By the time I left for Turkey, I was doing a T-Chart every week. And by the time I landed in Turkey, the things on my T-Chart that were once considered urgent were now labeled as secondary simply because at that point my secondary column just meant I was so used to the symptom that I hardly gave it a second thought; it was just how it was.

This T-Chart (Figure 4, page 30), recreated from one emailed to the doctor, is a huge leap from the one I made in September (See Figure 3, page 23), and it was only five months between the two. I felt like everything had accelerated in terms of the progression of scleroderma, and I wondered if this might have been triggered by the chemotherapy infusions we were doing to try and stop the progression. Or maybe things progressed because I had reached a point in my life where even my brain had gone on sick leave and I was no longer able to control things with my "mind over matter" mantra. But I do remember showing Dr. Gülbaş (the Turkish physician who would supervise my stem cell transplant) the slits in the corners of my mouth as we were walking into my rheumatologist's office for our consultation in Honolulu. He just shook his head and remained silent. Later during our appointment he told us that SCT was most successful in patients who were just in the beginning stages of the skin issues

URGENT	SECONDARY
Total Body Pain +20 every day	No energy
Difficulty taking deep breaths	Increased signs of CREST; especially Raynoud's
Diarrhea	No appetite
Vomiting after most meals	Tightening of skin on neck
Swallowing getting more difficult	Tightening and flaking of skin between fingers
Shortness of breath when walking Wheezing when going up one flight of stairs	
Increased rigidness in spine feels like knives being shoved into my torso on all sides	
Low grade fevers followed by low body temperature	
Low Blood Pressure	
Severe sweating when sleeping	
Tightening of skin around mouth with tears in each corner like very deep paper cuts in corner of my mouth	
Bleeding gums	

Figure 4: The pre-transplant T-Chart given to Dr. Gülbaş on February 15, 2011.

associated with scleroderma. I look at this list now and I think to myself, "How did I ever live like this?" but then I remember when Dr. Gülbaş looked at the same list, his response was one of hope. He read the list and assured me that SCT could handle it.

The next T-Chart, (Figure 5) also recreated from an email, shows were I was exactly one year post-transplant. Note the absence of symptoms like total body pain, difficulty swallowing, rigidness of spine, tightening of

URGENT	SECONDARY
Fatigue	Chemo-Induced Menopause
Chemo-Brain	Aseptic Necrosis
	Tendons and Trigger Fingers in Hands
	Bloody Nose
	Hay Fever

Figure 5: The T-Chart given to Dr. Gülbaş one year after the transplant, March 21, 2012.

skin—all symptoms of the autoimmune diseases that had been ravaging my body for so long. Gone. They're gone.

On the other hand, you'll notice two new symptoms on the right side of the chart. Both of these symptoms could have developed as part of my autoimmune diseases but they only emerged once the other more significant health symptoms subsided post-transplant. Both of these new symptoms affect the joints, with trigger finger obviously affecting the finger joints, and aseptic necrosis affecting hips, knees, and shoulders. Mine presented itself in my hips.

My quarterback was able to diagnose both symptoms through MRIs and we immediately moved into learning how to live with these symptoms. I started working right away with an occupational therapist. After consulting with Dr. Gülbaş about both issues I also learned something new. The chemotherapy and/or my autoimmune diseases may have caused trigger finger and aseptic necrosis, but because my transplant was successful I now have more good guy cells in my body. Consequently, there is the hope that as the new stem cells have a chance to grow and multiply there is the possibility that the aseptic necrosis could reverse itself, or at least slow its progress, and the trigger fingers could also become less frequent. As of the publication of this book, I am able to control any discomfort in my hips with ibuprofen. My trigger fingers are still quite painful, but I have a wide variety of custom made braces and the tools in place to relieve the pain as much as possible from my occupational therapist.

Maintaining my sensibility was a complicated task during the transplant phase. There were easy days where I didn't give a lot of thought to the isolation, the pain, the process, or the distance from home. There were hard days, though, and these would sorta pop up when I would least expect them. To clarify this point, I am going to share two stories—one of which I haven't been able to write about until this very moment while penning this chapter. The other story, well, we'll just say it is one of those that I just shoulda known. I'll start with the "shoulda known" story.

Menopause!? No matter if you are young or old, female or male, this word conjures up an image in your mind. It does for me, too. Most of us know that menopause happens as women get older; we know it is just part of life. What I shoulda known, and completely blanked on, is that menopause can be chemo induced. I should have remembered that when I had my hysterectomy, my OB/GYN mentioned that if I needed to have my ovaries removed or radiation or chemotherapy, I would experience chemo-induced menopause.

The major difference between normal menopause and chemotherapy-induced menopause is that the chemo-induced menopause happens immediately. No warning, no gradual onset, no chance to be slowly introduced to hot flashes. Nope, none of that; with chemo-induced menopause, I went from normal body temps (or normal for me) and in less than 24 hours after finishing the ATG (antithymocyte globulin) and Cytoxan infusions, I began to experience full-force internal combustion.

The next morning, after my first full night of hot flashes and night sweats every 20 to 30 minutes, Dr. Gülbaş came in for his daily rounds. He asked routine questions, but when he asked me if there was anything new I needed to tell him about. I said, "Yeah I'm having severe changes in my body temperatures every twenty to thirty minutes. I think my thermostat is broken." Dr. Gülbaş kind of chuckled and said that it was menopause. And I, being known for speaking my mind, said, "If I had known that menopause would feel like this and that it was a side effect of the SCT, I think I would not have agreed to one." Of course, my good sense soon returned, and I realized this would just be one side effect I would have to endure, and maybe I could just live with it—I mean, literally.

The second story I want to share is one that I have spent a lot of time pondering. I have tried many, many times over the past few years to get these thoughts onto paper. I might get two or three sentences written and then I would shut down. It was just too hard to remember and write. But now, I can.

On March 20, 2011, Dr. Gülbaş told me that the next morning, March 21, would be my "re-birth day." It would be the day that my stem cells would be injected back into my body. This was good news, of course. It was finally happening. The sooner I was transplanted and had engraftment (that is, when my stem cells began producing new cells), the sooner I could get out of the hospital and go home to Hawaii. Thinking along those lines kept me in tune with my sensibility and put into play all the information my partner Liz and I had learned about peripheral stem cell transplants. So, I was sensible enough to know that having made it to March 21, 2011, and having endured megadoses of total body eradication chemotherapy, my odds were better than good. I was in the home stretch and I was winning. This was, without doubt, being sensible.

However, as the hours ticked off the clock for March 20, 2011, so, too, was my normal commitment to sensibility. Dinner arrived at its normal 6:00 p.m., but by then I had no appetite. I felt trapped—stuck. Stuck in an isolation ward with no way to get in touch with anyone aside from Liz. With the time change everyone in my family was at home, in their beds, sleeping. I was here, in Turkey, far away from anything that resembled my home and I was wondering if I was actually going to die here. No, not just wondering if, but terrified that I would.

You see, chances of rejection or graft-versus-host disease (where the body attacks donor cells) are slim to none in autologous stem cell transplants. And in peripheral blood stem cell transplants, chances are even smaller. But it didn't matter. By 6:00 p.m. on the eve of my transplant, both my sense and my sensibility had abandoned me. The thought that kept racing through my mind, even when I was trying to sleep during the day, was what happens if my body rejects my own stem cells? And if that does happen, everything in my body has been wiped out so I can't even go back to living the way I had been, as bad as that was. Will I die fast? Will it be long and painful? Will I have enough time to talk to my parents, my brother and sister, my niece? I could not battle these thoughts; I could not shut them out.

They kept playing and replaying like the song you get stuck in your head and can't get rid of. Whenever I thought I had gotten through the gloom and doom, they would reappear. I didn't want my dinner; I didn't want to be bothered. Funny thing, though, was that on the outside, I appeared to just be going through another day in the transplant ward. Most days I was quiet and just kinda laid around so, on the outside, nothing seemed amiss. Liz wasn't aware that I was struggling with some pretty awful thoughts. That is, until she asked me some ordinary question, and I burst into tears. Not just tears, but all out crying and hysterical sobbing. There it was, out in the open; I was terrified. With everything that I knew about my illnesses, I should have remembered that experiencing this terror would be worth it if I were to have any chance at living. In rational moments of sensibility, I knew that my mental state was directly tied to my physical health, but I had to get beyond my irrational fear. Finally, I was sensible enough to know that talking about my feelings would help me to cope with them so I could be as ready as possible for March 21, 2011, my new birthday. Doesn't it just make sense that being a transplant patient would bring with it some fear?

Liz helped me get through that night. We used a lot of prayer and a lot of talking to accept that whatever lay ahead was really out of our hands.

The best way to show the impact of sensibility in the medical process is by looking at the second T-Chart (Figure 5, page 30) above and comparing it to the one before it (Figure 4, page 30)—the before and after record. Sensibility taught me to listen to my body and to pursue all avenues in order to get the treatment I needed. I really wish the FDA and insurance companies could use sensibility, too. I wonder what I might have spent on medical bills from 2011 through 2013 if I had not had the transplant. If I was able to live that long without the transplant, what would have been the cost of keeping me comfortable? What about the money I would have been entitled to through disability? How much money does an insurance company spend by denying a patient life-saving treatment? How much does the government spend in disability payments to patients who, with proper medical treatment, might no longer be disabled?

The cost of having my stem cell transplant in Turkey at a medical center with the same accreditation as the best hospitals in the United States was substantially less than all the medical expenses I had accumulated from 2005 through 2009. And that was just my co-pays. The cost of an uninsured transplant at home (if doctors were allowed to do it for cash) would have been $250,000. If the FDA permitted insurance companies to cover SCT in the U.S. and I had been able to get the SCT in my home state of Hawaii, our fundraising efforts would have easily covered the cost of the co-pays. But because I had to leave the country and travel halfway around the world, the cost effectively doubled. So going to a state-of-the-art facility in Turkey was a bargain at $56,000.

Chapter 3—Step2: Teamwork

"Coming together is a beginning. Keeping together is progress. Working together is success."
Henry Ford

Teamwork is a word all of us are familiar with. When someone uses the word around me, I always think back to the times in my life when I was part of a team—usually an athletic team: most particularly my high school soccer team and the high school girls' basketball team I coached, which were the ones that meant the most to me.

Have I heard the word teamwork used often on my medical journey? Actually, no. Teamwork isn't often thought to play a role in a patient's journey, at least when it involves the patient as the coach. Most commonly I would hear my doctors use the term to apply to the team of colleagues with whom they consult, with whom they share an office, and/or who assist in a procedure. To be fair to all past, present, and future health care providers, it's not surprising that the idea of the patient leading the team rarely occurred to my health care providers. In fact, it never occurred to me until one of my specialists, a dermatologist, mentioned it to me in 2008.

Perhaps I should back up to the year 1994 in my medical story and share a few details surrounding my health experiences as an adult. It was this background that propelled me to jump on the comment my dermatologist made: "You need to have a team of doctors where one doctor is the quarterback, and the others are the defensive line. And you need to be the coach."

Every year, with each new diagnosis, treatment, or procedure, I always thought to myself, "Okay, this is it. Once this is fixed I will feel good." And there were times between the ages of twenty-four and forty that I felt good. Or at least better than I had experienced before. For example, in 1994, I was led to my first GP in Maryland in search of why I was retaining fluid, why my abdomen was hard and tender, why I had major headaches that lasted for days, and why I was experiencing a major case of hives on the palms of my hands and soles of my feet. A number of diagnostic tests and procedures were recommended. I had my gall bladder removed and my left Achilles tendon repaired. It was much later that I learned that Achilles tendon issues are often associated with ankylosing spondylitis. (In 2003, I had my right Achilles tendon repaired.) After each procedure, I found some respite from daily pain, mostly due, I now believe, to the rest required for recovery.

Feeling good would last for a while, but ultimately old symptoms would return and new ones would appear, so back to the doctor I would go. Through the 1990s I believed that there was a routine path everyone should follow for their health care issues. First, you go to your GP, who would then recommend the next doctor, a specialist, for whatever testing needed to be completed. I had been conditioned to believe this—everything starts with your GP. Our societal structure had taught me that you have a pediatrician until you graduate to a GP, then you have an obstetrician/gynecologist (OB/GYN) for those "female" issues, and occasionally these doctors were supplemented by someone, for example, whom you regularly see for eye exams. Those were the big three in my world in the 1990s: GP, OB/GYN, and optician.

I believed that if I liked these doctors and felt comfortable with them, then everything would be fine because they definitely would stay on top of their craft. I was teaching full time by then, and I knew how stringent the local school district was about ensuring we teachers continually received professional development and worked toward our advanced degrees. Doctors did this too, right? This is what I was taught to believe. This is how I grew up.

However, I made the decision, as described in the previous chapter, to leave my GP and forge a new path to finding answers to what I had been told was "all in my head." I decided to go to one of the major university medical centers in my state, and fortunately (or unfortunately— however you want to see it) my symptoms were such that I was able to see a doctor who practiced both western and eastern medicine. What I found was that he was very interested in my health—specifically as it related to body, mind, and spirit. For him, it meant exploring both western and eastern approaches. If it meant trying acupuncture and homeopathic remedies, we tried that, too. What felt so refreshing was that this doctor never dismissed anything I said I was feeling. He would, then, become the quarterback for my team while I still lived in Maryland.

Through him I was directed to a specialist who ordered an MRI to measure the dissension of my cerebellar tonsils, which showed what is known as a "Chiari malformation." (I'll bet you didn't know we had tonsils in the back of our heads where they might or might not affect the brain stem!)

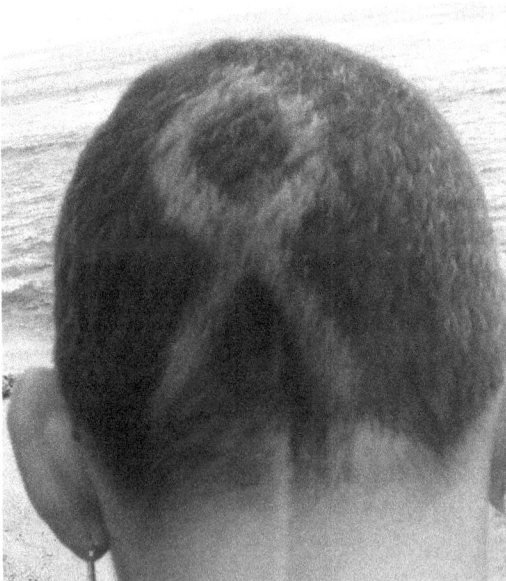

Post-transIplant, celebrating life with the green ribbon for stem cell/ bone marrow tranplant survivors. Note the scar at the nape of the neck-- it's from the Chiari malformation surgery.

Normally, the cerebellum and the brain stem sit in an indented space at the lower rear of the skull, above the opening to the spinal canal. When part of the cerebellum is located below this opening, it is called a Chiari malformation. Surgery to repair this problem involves making an incision at the back of the head and removing a small portion of the bottom of the skull to correct the irregular structure. The neurosurgeon uses a procedure that involves destroying tissue with high-frequency electrical currents, which shrinks the cerebellar tonsils. This is, by no means, a minor surgery.

Fortunately for me, my new quarterback—my eastern/ western/let's do what works doctor/quarterback—would support the decision to operate and repair this problem, but he also made sure my body, mind, and spirit were in the right place to recover quickly. This was the first time I experienced real teamwork in a medical setting. However, I was not the coach. I was still allowing the doctors to work as a team and fill me in on details after decisions for treatment were made. These were the early stages of my Step Two, Teamwork, which, at that time, still needed further development.

Although this was the beginning of what I would learn teamwork could mean, it was then that I began to realize that my medical care could be proactive versus reactive.

After my Chiari malformation repair (the brain stem surgery) in August of 2000, I began to feel completely different than I had ever felt. No headaches, no slurred speech, and best of all my swelling limbs and abdomen seemed to dissipate overnight. I was back to my happy size eight. I was feeling great, well, great by my standards. I still required a lot of rest and sleep, but I was ready to set out on one of the greatest adventures of my life. I was going to move 5,000 miles away from everything I've ever known in Maryland and set up my new home in Hawaii and begin my new job teaching at the university there.

I believed wholeheartedly that I wasn't going to be sick enough to warrant anything more than over-the-counter medications and my own doctoring. As all good children do when they leave home, I planned to return to my hometown twice a year (Christmas and summer) to see family and friends. And during those visits, even though I was on vacation, most of the people I wanted to visit worked full time so I could do my routine doctor appointments with all of the doctors I needed to see. This would allow me to avoid finding doctors in Honolulu because, of course, after the brain stem surgery, I seriously believed that those mild symptoms I still experienced were not affecting my daily life—at least not significantly. On my trips back to Maryland I planned to do my dental visits, my annual GYN exam, and my eye exam.

I moved to Hawaii on July 7, 2004. I returned to Maryland for Christmas that same December and stayed until January 4, 2005. I had three doctor's appointments scheduled (dentist, GYN, and eye), and it would be the routine visit to my longstanding gynecologist that would change my world, medically speaking. I had been going to him since I was eighteen and I knew the office staff, nurses, and all of the doctors. I felt comfortable there. The doctor was also a great friend of my mom, who had worked with him in the operating room since he had graduated from medical school. There was nothing unusual about the exam—everything seemed fine according to the doctor. We talked a lot about my new job and home. It was by all accounts the same kind of visit I had had with this doctor in this office for the past sixteen years. When I say by all accounts, I mean nothing appeared different, absolutely nothing. I wasn't having any pain. I hadn't missed a period. And I had never, ever had an abnormal Pap smear.

About two weeks after returning to Hawaii and starting the spring semester, I arrived home to a message on my answering machine from my doctor in Maryland asking me to call him back. It was too late to call that day, since we are six hours behind in Hawaii, so I dismissed the thought and put it on my to-do list for the following morning. Later that evening, I talked with my mother who asked if I had heard anything from my GYN. I said I had gotten a message but hadn't had time to return it. I asked why she brought it up and she said that the doctor had called her to verify my phone number in Hawaii. I could sense something was awry by my mom's tone. But when I pressed her on the issue, all she could say was that when she asked the doctor if everything was all right, he said he needed to talk with me first. In hindsight, I appreciate that he respected the doctor/patient relationship and waited to discuss the situation with me first. Because he knew my mom so well, and because she had worked with him, he could have decided to give her the information, but his professionalism won out and for that I am grateful.

I did make contact with him the following day. He delivered the news I did not want to hear: "We have the results of your Pap smear and it has come back positive for adenocarcinoma." He continued, "I was so shocked by the result that I had the smear sent to another testing facility for a second opinion, and that result came back positive, too." My first reaction, "Okay. What is adenocarcinoma?" He explained as carefully as he could. I could tell he was upset at having to tell me this news over the phone across so many miles. He kept asking me if I was okay and apologizing. Me, well, I just kept saying the "C" word.

Then it dawned on me that my sister had had several abnormal Pap smears and they just monitored and watched for further changes. I decided that was what he would tell me. While all of this was spinning in my head, I knew my doctor was still talking on the other end of the phone line, but I wasn't exactly listening to him. Finally I was jolted back into reality when he said, quite firmly, "Cristy, I need you to repeat back to me what you need to do next." I fessed up that I had no idea what he had said, so he explained that I needed to see a doctor right away. I had two choices, get on a plane that night and fly back to Maryland to see him or spin the roulette wheel to find a gynecologist in Honolulu. Flying home was not an option. Before I knew it my team of doctors was about to change as my location dictated the need for a new doctor right away.

Cancer. I was scared and I had no time to waste. I got on the Internet right away and started surfing for a gynecological oncologist in Honolulu. After researching women's cancer centers in Honolulu, I selected an oncologist affiliated with Kapiolani Women's and Children Center. I called the doctor's office and explained to the receptionist my situation. She told me that the oncologist only saw patients after the diagnosis was confirmed and they require a referral from an OB/GYN. My heart sank in the moment of silence after her words. Amazingly, she could have dismissed me right then and there, but instead she asked me to hold on for a second. When she came back to the phone she told me she spoke with the doctor and his nurse, both of whom gave her the name of the same GYN.

With no other guidance to go on, I called this doctor. By the grace of God, I had made a good choice. I explained my situation to the receptionist: that I had just moved to Hawaii and just found out my Pap smear results from a test done in Maryland. Instead of telling me the doctor was not accepting new patients, she placed me on hold and went to talk to his nurse. The nurse got on the line and I described my situation again and told her my doctor in Maryland was so shocked by the results of my Pap smear that he had sent it to two different labs. The nurse placed me hold for less than a minute and when she got back on the line she told me the doctor would see me the next morning at ten o'clock. I breathed a long sigh of relief, but at the same time, I knew that the immediacy of the appointment meant this was bad—this was very bad. The appointment the following morning led to two surgeries.

My cancer had started in the uterus and pelvic wall and spread to the cervix, where the Pap smear picked it up. Oddly enough, I had no symptoms and did not test positive for human papilloma virus, which is common in this cancer. First, the doctor performed what is called a conization, or cone biopsy, which confirmed I had Stage 3 cancer and provided information regarding how extensive the hysterectomy would need to be. Six weeks later, I had the hysterectomy. The success of these surgeries mean that, among other things, I am now a cancer survivor. I never, for a moment, thought that I would subsequently survive a great deal more than cancer.

After my hysterectomy (2005), I never felt quite right. Things in my body just didn't go back to the way things felt prior to surgery. Actually, I began to experience symptoms similar to those I had leading up to the Chiari malformation repair.

In 2006, I had surgery to repair a Meckel's Diverticulum along with an intestinal resection to remove a cancerous growth which was discovered during the endoscopy. Again, I hoped these procedures would relieve many of the strange symptoms I was experiencing, but it didn't happen. I had the feeling that there was something more going on in my body besides the issues that had been addressed. Nothing felt right after that. There had to be something else.

Some of those symptoms from 1994 returned. I was retaining fluid in my hands and feet, having difficulty swallowing, and developing hive-like bumps on my arms and hands. Had the repair failed? Have I developed syringomyelia (cysts or tumors that form in the spinal cord— something I had read about when researching the Chiari malformation surgery)? If it had been something else all along, was the brain stem surgery a waste of time? I began doubting myself and the need for Chiari malformation repair and sometimes wondered if my GP from Maryland was right, that I really was a hypochondriac.

But after thinking deeply about it, I decided that I was not a hypochondriac and I refused to allow myself to go into that dark hopelessness; I refused to believe it or even think it. There was something else wrong and whether it had anything to do with a previous surgery, I didn't know, but by damn I was going to find out. Whatever was happening, whatever was going on with my body, I would pursue these health issues until I found answers. I was an adult with my own health insurance, living on my own, and I was the only person who was going to make decisions for me. I became a person on a mission and I was going to get to the heart of my health symptoms once and for all so I could make good decisions.

Finding the new GYN in Honolulu brought with it more than I could have imagined. Through him I found a new GP and eventually created the team of physicians who currently "play for me."

The Team

I need to preface this section by telling you that any team you assemble MUST change over time as your needs change. The makeup of your team must be organic, changing from time to time in order to respond to your changing needs. This is especially important if you have issues like mine, issues that don't lead to a single diagnosis and treatment protocol. When you are suffering from so many different medical problems, the results of diagnostic testing are often contradictory and inconclusive. I have confidence that the physicians with whom you work will have your best interests in mind and will understand any need for change.

I want to share with you the most effective ways to let go of certain doctors and the best ways to add new members to your team. Ultimately it is the coach who pencils in the starting lineup, determines who will be sitting on the bench for the time being, and who may, in fact, need to be retired or traded.

I am the coach of my team and you are the coach of yours. When your needs or your physical condition changes, the lineup—or even the makeup of the team—must change. In 2008, when my dermatologist suggested that I needed a team, he explained that I had to be the coach and I had to have a quarterback, a defensive line, and an offensive line to work with me, who, through cooperation, would bring their best skills to bear in the contest against my medical problems. Maybe the quarterback would be calling the plays most of the time, but he, and the rest of the defensive line, would include me in all decisions regarding treatment options. They would not work around me; they would work for me.

I should say, though, that your success at building such a team and being recognized and respected as the coach is dependent on how well you educate yourself about your medical issues. Most doctors appreciate well-informed patients; they appreciate being pointed into directions they may not have considered. You are the expert on you, remember? Share your expertise with your doctors.

What follows is the story of how my first medical team in Hawaii came into existence, how it has changed over time, who is currently on the roster, and how it may change in the future.

I am the coach. I will always be the coach. Even as I write this, I feel empowered, and you, also, will feel that way. There is something liberating about taking charge of your health care. There is something else I did that you need to take into consideration: even if my health is such that I cannot speak or act for myself, I have put into place the pieces of the game plan that can be carried out by my team in case I am "ejected" for any reason. (I am proud to say I was never ejected or given a technical foul while coaching high school sports. In the case of my medical care, I will gladly allow myself to be ejected or served a foul if it means my body, mind and spirit gets what it needs. Within reason, of course.) You, too, must make provisions for those times when you may not be able to direct your team.

Positions on My Team

Quarterback: This player calls the plays in consultation with the coach, keeping other members of the team informed, and is willing to invest in the coach's game plan. The quarterback has the ability to form a new patient/doctor relationship that involves communicating in non-traditional ways to avoid wasting face-to-face appointment time. The quarterback is willing to look outside the box and consult members of the offensive line when the coach feels it is necessary. The quarterback is able to assess input from the starting members of the defensive line, as well as the offensive line, and make recommendations. Because Liz went with me to every appointment, she contributed considerable information regarding my day-to-day progress, keeping lines of communication open for the quarterback to the offensive line.

Defensive Line: The medical professionals (including office support staff and nurses) who are receptive to the calls of the quarterback make up the defensive line. They provide expertise in their specialties, work tirelessly to defend against progression of the diseases, help treat the symptoms, seek proactive treatment options, and remain open to thinking outside of the box. The defensive line receives medical updates from all other team players following appointments and diagnostic testing. They also receive and file all diagnostic test results.

Offensive Line: This is my *'ohana*. In Hawaiian culture, it means family (in an extended sense of the term, which goes beyond blood relationships to adoptive and intentional or voluntary members of a family group). The concept emphasizes that families are bound together and members must cooperate and "remember one another;" that is, that nobody gets left behind. My *'ohana* includes friends, family, supporters, and donors, some of whom I don't even know, who stood with me and never gave up on my fight for treatment. They were my cheerleaders and my fans, sitting in the bleachers or watching the contest from afar. They stood with me in my search for medical care no matter where in the world that would be. My *'ohana* are the folks who still raise me up, while at the same time keeping me grounded. They allow me to practice my faith and keep my mission going even after the stem cell transplant was done and I moved on to learning to live. They are still with me and still supporting me in ways too numerous to count.

Being your own patient advocate is something that continues even after the treatment has been administered.

It is my *'ohana* that continues to keep me going, just as they did at those times when I felt like giving up or giving in to so many pressures. There were times when it would have been easy to throw my hands up, file for disability, and settle into a dark, quiet place and await death, but my *'ohana* reminded me of my purpose in this life. They pushed me to recognize a purpose from which others would learn by my example and fight to survive.

Look around you. Who is your *'ohana*? Who are the people who will be there when you need them to lift you up and keep you going? Later in this chapter, I will share more about my *'ohana* and what they did that helped me through such a difficult time.

The Bench: These are the specialty players, those medical professionals who are essential to my care, but not necessarily on a regular basis. For example, my neurologist is still on my team, but once it was determined that my illnesses/symptoms were not related to Chiari malformation, he was moved to second string. He is a wonderful doctor and exceptional in his trade. Should the need for a neurologist arise anywhere in my future, I will put him in the game.

How I Use My Team

The quarterback is my rheumatologist, Dr. Kristine M. Uramoto. It turned out that my major health issues were all related to autoimmune diseases. Simply put, an autoimmune disease is the result of your body's natural protection against disease gone wrong. Our immune system is designed to help protect the body against harmful agents by producing antibodies that destroy the harmful agents. Unfortunately, there are times when the body gets confused and begins to send antibodies to attack perfectly healthy body tissues. Nobody seems to know why this short-circuit happens, but it happens and sometimes it is deadly.

We often think of the rheumatologist as someone who treats common conditions like arthritis, but because autoimmune diseases attack bodily tissue, a rheumatologist is often called upon to treat a variety of autoimmune diseases. So it would be the easy choice to select her as my quarterback. But, more importantly, she is the quarterback because of how our doctor/patient relationship was built on mutual respect with a mutual goal.

My medical journey didn't start out this way. In 2006, I was filtering everything through my GP with the expectation that he could take all of my issues and then refer me to the appropriate specialist for follow up or further testing. For some people, their GP is a good choice for quarterback. In my situation, my GP was not an expert in rheumatologic illnesses. Nor was he able to spend the amount of time with me during office visits to adequately investigate all possible causes. This does not mean he is a bad doctor or not qualified as a GP. He is one of the best. But like most GPs he is overworked and understaffed. What my GP did for me, which gave me more than anything else, was to connect me with other doctors who could do what he couldn't. My GP gave me the permission I needed to seek help from specialists, while he was willing to stay on the team, even if it meant not always being a starter.

The strongest team I have ever assembled began playing together in 2008. It would culminate with the addition of a new playing field near Istanbul, Turkey, and then a new set of starters for the team in Hawaii post-transplant.

Hawaii Medical Team—My Defensive Line

Specialty	Dates	Team Status
*General Practitioner	2006-Present	Starter
*Rheumatologist	2006–Present	Starter/Quarterback
*Gastroenterologist	2006-2007	Starter
Gastroenterologist	2006-2008	Waiting on the bench

Colorectal Surgeon	2005-2006	Available, if needed
General Surgery	2006	Waiting on the bench
*Dermatologist	2006-Present	Starter
*Eyes	2007-2011	Available, if needed
*OB/GYN	2005-Present	Starter
*Psychiatrist	2006-2013	Waiting on the bench
Neuropsychologist	2013-Present	Starter
Psychiatrist	2013-Present	Starter
Occupational Therapy	2013-Present	Starter
*Cardiologist	2007-Present	Starter
Ear, Nose, and Throat	2016-1010	Available, if needed
Neurologist	2006-2010	Available, if needed
*Pain Management	2009-2011	Available, if needed
Pulmonologist	2007-2012	Waiting on the bench
*Cardiologist	2007-Present	Waiting on the bench
*Represents my strongest Hawaii team to date		

You will note that some of my strongest players are not necessarily in the starting lineup (at this writing). Some are on the bench, and some are waiting somewhere off the playing field. The important thing to know about these players is that where they are at any given moment is okay with them—they understand their roles.

Recruitment began in 2006, but the full team wasn't functioning until 2008, after receiving a confirmed set of diagnoses (scleroderma, ankylosing spondylitis, and vasculitis) and a second opinion from Mayo Clinic, Scottsdale. Missing from the chart are the most important members of the team, aside from the quarterback (my rheumatologist), which is my offensive line.

My Offensive Line

My offensive line consists of my *'ohana*, the people who know me, care about me, and are always there to carry the coach when I couldn't carry myself.

My offensive line fell into place in a very strange way in 2008. I was working with an educational consulting team from the University of Hawaii in Guam, where I had to live with other people 24/7 for two weeks. As a result, I could no longer hide my pain and health struggles. For example, it is very hard to hide the fact that you are giving yourself methotrexate injections in the abdomen every week or to keep a low profile when you have to take out your needles, syringes, and little vials of vital chemo-based drugs when checking through the security line at the airport.

I also couldn't hide the fact that I was living off of $40.00 per week for food and any other items I needed. Forty dollars is all that I had left each week after paying my monthly minimums on credit cards (used for medical co-pays, fees for diagnostic testing, and prescription co-pays) along with other required bills we all have (like car insurance, gas, rent). It was there, in Guam, that my friends (my budding 'ohana) would develop the idea of putting together a fundraiser with the hope of paying off a quickly growing mountain of medical debt. The work of this group of educational consultants on my behalf led to new hope in ways I could have never imagined.

That first fundraiser turned out to be more than a fund-raising effort. It was there that I met the woman who would become my partner, Liz. The event was held at the Episcopal Church, The Parish of St. Clement, in Honolulu, where she is the priest. When I met her, I knew that I had I found my soul mate, and, not surprisingly, my loudest cheerleader. The details of our relationship aren't relevant to this particular book, but it is important to know that Liz was willing to give up everything in her life to accompany me on my medical journey from that moment on, even, when the time came, going with me to Turkey for my stem cell transplant. Her love sustained me through the transplant as she made the choice to enter isolation with me so I would not have to face it alone.

Over the next few months Liz would reach out to other members of the community—those who would eventually

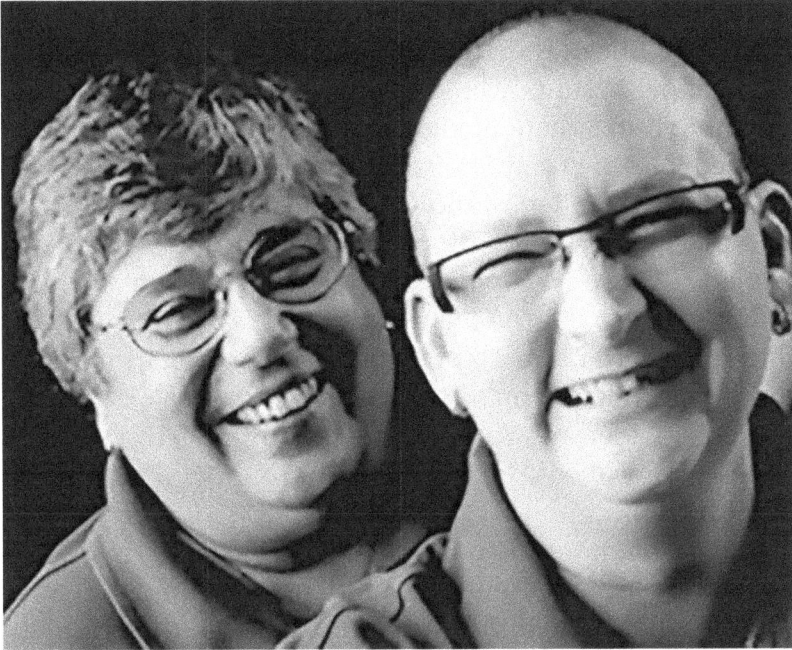

Liz and Cristy, post-transplant

join the offensive line, those who were to become *'ohana* to me even if not through blood, and the wheels started turning for what would eventually be known as the *One of Our Own Fund*.

The *One of Our Own Fund* started out with a small group of my *'ohana* who believed that we should cast a wider net to find sources of funding for my medical care, which, it became increasingly clear, would be extremely expensive. Through email conversations with Liz, some of my colleagues from the University of Hawaii, and long-time friend, Sharon Miller, the *One of Our Own Fund* took on a life of its own with a website, a board of directors, and an organized fund-raising strategy. And so, by the end of 2009, the offensive line was in full force with a successful fund-raising effort that cast its net beyond local events into cyberspace and across the mainland.

As my *'ohana* considered the possibilities for the future of the *One of Our Own Fund* website and organization, they believed that they could create a model for others who might have the need or the desire to raise money for one of their own, for someone with unrelenting medical debt and nowhere else to turn, and to perpetuate the model for others along the way. With that hope, they applied for 501c3 status with the Internal Revenue Service, through which they would help other local groups set up a similar structure. Unfortunately, the application was denied because it only benefited a single person. The IRS didn't seem to get the idea of paying it forward and how the exponential growth of such a network could multiply the support for people who needed financial assistance across a wider network. In the meantime, though, the state of Hawaii did recognize the group as a non-profit organization.

My *'ohana* was bound and determined to find a way to raise the money I would need to find a doctor somewhere in the world who would do the peripheral stem cell transplant—something that we then knew was the only hope since such a procedure was not and would never be available here in the United States—at least not in my lifetime (which was looking shorter every day). The single, most important thing my offensive line did for me was remove me from the fund-raising process. This allowed me to focus on staying as healthy as I could and working with my medical team until I found a transplant doctor. Moreover, it relieved me of the stress of feeling like I was begging people for money.

I need to make mention of the fact that, for you, the players on the offensive line will also change over time. This is one of the hardest parts of any medical journey because it is the offensive line players to whom we are personally closest. These players are most often our family members, our friends (some dating back for decades), spouses/partners, and colleagues that we see on a daily basis.

To be completely honest, my offensive line, during the transplant in 2011, looked very little like my offensive line in 2007. It's not always easy to know why it changes. Is it because some of these players were worn out by all the medical drama? Were they tired of me not being able to get up and go when they needed something or wanted to do something? Could it be that sometimes I let my barriers down and they saw me in some of my worst times of pain and vulnerability and other times they saw me "perform" for a class I taught or meeting I was attending so they wondered if I was faking it?

If I had a penny for every time someone said to me, "You look fine, you must be fine," I wouldn't have any medical debt at all. Truth be told, I was a master manipulator. I lived with pain for so long and had conditioned myself to believe the mantra of "No pain, no gain," that there were times I could be in public that I, too, would forget I was experiencing a severe health crisis. For example, I was so good, in fact, that I returned to teach class just two weeks after my hysterectomy, catheter and all. But as soon as I returned to the safety of my home and allowed myself to sit down and relax, the pain would all come flooding back.

Remember when I wrote that I had been to a doctor in Maryland who used both western and eastern medical approaches? The lessons he taught me I still practice today. Lessons such as total body meditation and relaxation and the ability to use mind over matter. I actually learned the process of visual meditation from my high school soccer coach. It worked so well for me that I taught it to my players when I coached high school basketball. Because I could do these things, sometimes I could mask the most overt symptoms, which made some people doubt me.

The flip side of this is what my health did to me in terms of my mind, or how I interacted with people. There were times, after thirty-plus years of dealing with and coping with pain, that I wasn't always pleasant to those who were closest to me. There were times I was mean, angry, or just so tired that one little comment would set me off. I have several regrets about this and I know some of those relationships will never be repaired. All I can do, then, is to work honestly with my therapist and talk about triggers that make me act that way and focus on how to avoid hurting those close to me. I have not perfected this yet, but I still actively work on the "who" I want to be. I know that part of this journey is adapting to my new "normal" and learning how to live. Since my transplant, I have reached out to some of these people and acknowledged my bad behavior and apologized.

Dealing with Change on the Offensive Line

I wish I could tell you to just forget the players on the offensive line who don't support you, by either questioning your health care choices, always one-upping you, or flat out questioning if you are sick at all. I wish I could say that I just decided to bench these players and move on to a stronger offensive line. But I didn't always do that. For a long time I listened to their questions and tried to answer sincerely when they asked how I was feeling; too often, though, before I could finish one complete sentence I would be cut off so they could share their personal drama, or I could just oblige them when they said, "You look fine. C'mon, let's go do...."

I even conditioned myself to use key phrases around certain people so I would never have to share my real thoughts regarding how I was on that day or what I had been up to that had kept me away or busy. Instead of saying something like, "I had three doctor's appointments this week, a CAT scan, and an MRI," I would say, "I was busy with work."

Eventually as time and my deteriorating health took its toll, my offensive line was thinned out due to things beyond my control. What I mean is that by late 2010, I was on 'round the clock morphine tablets and Vicodin. So I spent upwards of fourteen hours a day sleeping. If I wasn't calling or emailing folks on my offensive line, they weren't calling or emailing me, either. Once, a former player on my offensive team called to ask me out to lunch. She said that she could meet me near my house or somewhere in town. I told her I had moved to Hawaii Kai (twelve miles away) and wasn't driving much. Her reply was, "Well, I'm not driving that far for lunch." She didn't get it, and I didn't have the energy to explain it. I'm sure she thought I was brushing her off.

Sometimes I find myself missing some of my closest friends. And I'm still sad for the good times which are no more. I still get upset that they aren't around; I cared a lot for them, but I failed to make them see what was happening to me. They didn't respond to emails I sent during my transplant in Turkey (making phone calls was impossible due to time change and sleeping schedule), or, when they were notified of fund-raising events, they either didn't realize the seriousness of my diseases or they questioned my honesty. It makes me sad, but I can't dwell on it. I'm sorry, but a person doesn't voluntarily sign up for chemo infusions every three weeks unless something is really, really wrong. And last time I checked, to get Rituxan infusions you need a doctor's prescription.

You see what I've just done? I just spent too much time focusing on something negative by describing the difficulty of dealing with some of the changes in my offensive line. But you have to be prepared for it; your offensive line will change over time. Maybe not because you want it to, but because health care issues have a way of weeding out those who may call you friend, but really can't see beyond how your friendship is a benefit to them.

In retrospect, though, I can see both sides of this issue. There were times that I was probably short with some friends who didn't really know what I was up against. If I want to repair any of those friendships, it needs to be me who takes the first step. I will do my best to make amends.

Creating the Team

The mantra for this section is, "It is always the coach's decision." We have been taught to believe that doctors can be trusted to know what they are doing. We also look toward family, friends, or colleagues to recommend good doctors. But what fits for someone else may not be the right fit for you. You are the coach. Do not assume that your discomfort with your doctor will change over time, that it will get better. The only way the doctor/patient relationship will grow is if there is a level of mutual respect and comfort from the very instant you meet.

As my mother used to tell me when she took me shoe shopping for school, "If it doesn't feel right or fit when you first try it on, you won't wear them. So don't waste my money." If something feels "off," or you just don't feel heard or comfortable the first time you meet your doctor, don't waste your money and go back. This also applies if initially you build rapport with your doctor then something happens that makes you uncomfortable. You (or your insurance company if you are lucky) are paying for your doctor's expertise and service. In return you should expect to be heard and cared for. A good example of this was when, in 2006, I was referred to a surgeon for my Meckel's repair and small intestine resection. The second I entered the doctor's office, the nurse began gushing in a too-familiar way that did not seem, in any way, sincere. She started talking to me like she was my BFF (best friend forever in current textspeak), asking me if I had plans for the weekend and giving me her opinion about a recent state political issue. It was weird. I am used to having office staff being friendly and making me feel welcome, but I have never discussed politics with anyone on my medical team. (Oh, yes, I have, but only to debate the stem cell transplant possibilities and the fact that a peripheral stem cell transplant does not impact anyone but me; therefore, the choice should be mine.) In hindsight, I should have walked out of that office and never looked back. But I, too, did what many of us do, thinking, "she certainly doesn't reflect the expertise of the doctor." FACT: Never underestimate the power the office staff has over a doctor's practice. In the case of this particular doctor, I should have listened to my gut instead of convincing myself to go through with the surgery.

When I arrived at the hospital the day of the operation, the hospital had me scheduled for check in because I would be staying overnight, but the doctor's nurse had failed to notify the operating room scheduler that I was on his surgical calendar for that day. The nurse also forgot to write it into the office calendar so the doctor would know his own schedule. When I arrived, he was already in surgery with another patient and had a full day of procedures scheduled. When the OR staff informed him I was there and the scheduling snafu was result of his staff's error, he left his current surgical patient (just cut open on the table??) to chat with me. He assured me he could "squeeze" me in between other patients. FACT: it is never too late to change or reschedule medical procedures or treatment if your gut or heart is not in it. In hindsight this is the second opportunity I had to walk away from this doctor and I didn't. Looking back, I wish I had. I still am suffering side effects from a procedure that most likely was "sequenced" into a schedule. And by the way, this doctor was dismissed from my team permanently two months after surgery.

A solid, strong, professional relationship with a doctor does not mean getting a discount. It does not mean going out for drinks or other social activities. It does not mean the doctor agrees with or supports you on every test, medication or diagnosis you suggest. It does not necessarily mean calling each other by your first names (sometimes this does happen, but usually it is not a forced dynamic but rather one that just seems to fall into place). A solid, strong, professional relationship between a doctor and patient is built on mutual respect; the respect you have for the doctor's knowledge and skills AND the respect your doctor has for you and your intelligence. From the very first second you meet your doctor, there should be a level of comfort in knowing that the doctor is asking thoughtful, caring, probing questions and listens to you as you share.

This is where the T-Chart comes in handy. (See Chapter 2.) Your T-charts will keep the conversation on track. For the first two years I was seeing my rheumatologist, I did not try to engage with her outside of office appointments. If I had been doing research on the Internet or found some new diagnosis that fit my symptoms, I made sure to call her office and schedule an appointment. It was only after two years of working with her (my quarterback) that we mutually agreed that there would be some benefit to communicating via email. This, of course, does not work in cases of emergencies. Email does, however, alleviate the need block off a forty-five minute appointment time where I am just handing her new information on research studies in the United States, or new treatment options for scleroderma, vasculitis, and ankylosing spondylitis. Email gave my doctor more time for patients who need the face-to-face visit and she could read the information we were discussing at a time when her schedule permitted. It also freed me from the added burden of another appointment to add to my already crowded schedule. (By 2009, I was going to at least one doctor's appointment per week, and often seeing the starting line up every month.)

Technology has changed since I started my medical journey, and I am sure if I were still in pre-transplant phase, my quarterback and I would have also texted to one another. Regardless of how you communicate with your quarterback, one very important thing to remember is that each of you needs to respect each other's personal email addresses, phone numbers, and social media outlets. Meaning, do not start forwarding emails to your doctor (even if you think it's the funniest joke in history), do not give out personal contact information to anyone, and do not sign them up for product notices or discussion groups.

Your Medical Team MUST Change Over Time

As I mentioned before, you have to realize that your team MUST change over time. Health issues are not stagnant. Even diseases that are diagnosed, treated and cured, or are in remission, leave the patient with after effects that still require medical follow up. As symptoms change, the team players have to change to address those changes.

Early in my medical journey in Hawaii, one of the major symptoms I experienced was fatigue. This is still a major symptom in my life, and probably always will be, but in 2006, we had not been able to attribute it to a specific cause. My GP, in good form, referred me to an endocrinologist. This was the right referral for the time. But once we determined my symptoms were not linked to my endocrine system, there was no longer a need for an endocrinologist to be in the starting lineup. He was moved to the bench.

Fatigue has never been a symptom I have been able to get a handle on, but the causes for it have changed post-transplant. Pre-transplant fatigue was associated with my diseases and their treatment (including prescription pills, methotrexate injections and chemotherapy infusions of cytoxan and Rituxan), along with a rigorous work schedule (necessary to receive promotion and tenure at the university so I could keep my job, my health insurance, as well as take advantage of my sick leave). Because of this, my starting lineup included a pain management specialist who oversaw all possible side effects from the different drugs and also prescribed some medications to help keep me alert enough to work. Once I returned home in 2011 after the transplant, I no longer needed him in my starting lineup. I am happy to report that I am only on over-the-counter (OTC) maintenance medication now (Zyrtec, Prilosec), along with a prescription antidepressant, and the occasional antibiotic for a cold or sinus infection.

Post-transplant, my fatigue directly correlates to the trauma my body endured during the transplant. You may not know that there are four major stages of the stem cell transplant process. Let me try to simplify it for you. First, you undergo a course of chemotherapy, which is designed to depress your immune system. Second, your stem cells are harvested from your body. This is something like dialysis where a machine draws your blood out of one arm, passes it through a "magic" machine which extracts the stem cells from the blood, and then returns the remaining blood components back into your body through the other arm. This process can take up to six hours and may need to be done over multiple days until a sufficient number of stem cells are collected. Third, you are hit again with another, even more powerful, course of chemotherapy which is designed to completely kill off your immune system—you know, that part of you that is trying to kill you? Finally, the stem cells are transfused through a shunt in your neck that sends the cells directly into your heart for rapid deployment throughout your body.

Think about it. They had to kill my immune system. When a baby is born, it has the benefit of its mother's antibodies until the baby begins to produce its own antibodies and its immune system takes over from mama. In order for my reconditioned stem cells to take hold and multiply as new, healthy stem cells, everything else in my body had to be shut down. I wouldn't have the benefit of any protective immunity until my stem cells rebuilt my immune system and began building new cells, something that

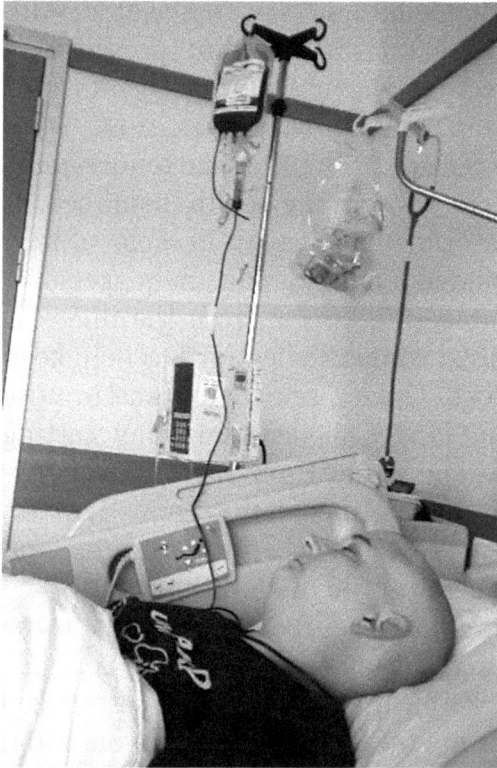

The dark area in the transfusion bag is a cloud of Cristy's very own stem cells, ready to go to work for her.

would take me longer than it takes a newborn baby. The risk of infection after this procedure is extremely high. Today, I celebrate March 21, 2011, as my new birthday. It is the day I was reborn.

Chemotherapy brings its own menu of severe and unpleasant side effects, and the amount of total body eradication chemotherapy used in a stem cell or bone marrow transplant is astonishing. One of my technicians in Turkey compared the amount of chemotherapy that I received in one week to the amount of chemotherapy a breast cancer patient may receive over five years of treatment.

My gastroenterologist likes to compare a stem cell transplant to his favorite kinds of movies, with the classic battle of good versus evil. The stem cells are the heroes called in to save the day after the chemotherapy (the bad guy) has almost destroyed, or wiped out, an entire civilization. This is a very close analogy, except in the prequel to this movie, the chemotherapy was the good guy unloading his entire arsenal on an enemy even more dangerous than he. It is later that the stem cells come along to make certain that the chemotherapy doesn't let power go to his head.

Perhaps I've taken the long way around just to identify my starting lineup post-transplant. Two years post-transplant, I became very concerned about cognitive issues. Among other things, I was having trouble concentrating for any length of time. I discovered this is not unusual after such a massive dose of chemotherapy; I call it "chemo-brain." Fatigue continued to be a problem so I added a neuro-psychologist to my starting defensive line and now she oversees the fatigue and cognitive rehabilitation.

Prior to getting my stem cell transplant, I was waiting to die. Having all of my cognitive abilities or needing to be awake to work wasn't high on my list of priorities. I hope the effects were not long lasting. Post-transplant, being free of symptoms of autoimmune diseases has forced me to learn how to live. This means I need to learn to think again and also to build recovery time into my daily schedule. Without this, my fatigue can be all consuming.

How to Let Go of Players and Move On

Have you ever had a doctor tell you they have reached the limit of their medical expertise? This may be rare, but it does happen. In the case of my first gastroenterologist, he was at a loss after I had been officially diagnosed with scleroderma and the FDA pulled the medication I needed off the market. I needed this medication to make my esophagus contract so I could swallow. This is far more serious than acid reflux or heartburn and medications routinely prescribed for those conditions were of no use. My esophagus was not functioning; food could not move through it.

This doctor had stood with me for quite a while as I searched for a diagnosis or diagnoses; he worked well with my quarterback (rheumatologist), and he even supported the decision to seek a second opinion from the Mayo Clinic. It was the Mayo Clinic which, through esophageal dysmotility testing, confirmed his suspicion: 60% of the time my esophagus did not contract during swallowing. And once the medication I needed was removed from the market in the United States, this doctor did not know what else to do for me. During an office visit, we talked about mail order medications from outside the U.S. and the problem of not knowing if they have been manufactured safely with accurate ingredients; we talked about pace makers for the esophagus; and he suggested I consider talking with other gastroenterologists who may know a bit more about esophageal problems associated with scleroderma.

This doctor made my coaching decision for me. He even had his office manager call and set up an appointment for me with another gastroenterologist down the street. For him, my healthcare wasn't about how much money he could make but rather his own self-awareness that my condition had exceeded his knowledge base, and that he wouldn't have time to do independent research to find alternative methods of treatment. He knew he needed to retire from the team. He made a hard decision easy.

This isn't always the case. Sometimes as the coach, and largest stakeholder in the team, we must sit a player or trade a player, that is, a doctor on the defensive line. We have to make the very hard decision. The best way I know to explain this is to share a story about the hardest decision I've ever had to make regarding a doctor.

In 2007, I lost my best friend, my buddy, singer and performer, Don Ho (my relationship with Don could be a book or movie all by itself). His death affected me in a way that I had never experienced. Realizing I was suffering from depression, I sought help from a psychiatrist. Depression was only one concern, as you might guess. Navigating the medical maze and spending most of my time dealing with physical issues inevitably led to what I believed were emotional and mental issues. After years of being sick and trying to hide my pain from others, I needed an antidepressant to keep me going and I needed someone

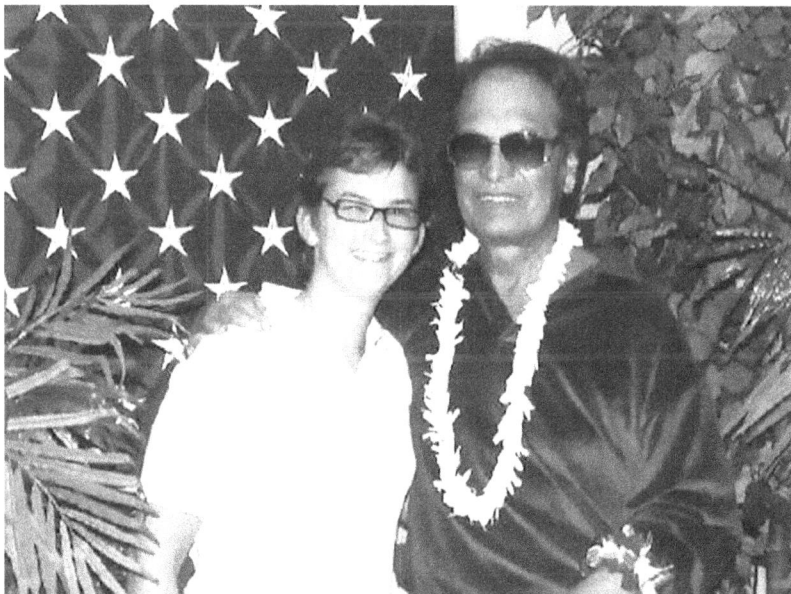

Cristy with Don Ho, 2006

that I could talk to about the fact I spent most of my life hiding how I was really feeling physically.

From the time I had met Don in 1999, he was fully aware of my health issues. In fact, Don Ho was my only visitor when I was hospitalized for my hysterectomy (2005). To me, Don was the one person who could read me without my ever having to say a word. He knew my pain and he understood why I needed to carry on in my life and career hiding as much as I could from colleagues and acquaintances. As a single female living 5,000 miles from home, he understood my need to appear strong, and he knew illness was often seen as weakness.

In my estimation, Don Ho was a medical pioneer and a role model. His determination and will to live pushed him to seek medical options outside of the U.S. to help cure his heart condition. FDA regulations deemed him unsuitable for a heart transplant or any other type of experimental heart procedure being conducted in the United States. Because there was increasing talk in the medical community of stem cell transplants as a means of resolving multiple medical issues, Don set out to find a way to get stem cells for his heart. The idea of medical tourism as a viable health care option only crossed my radar because Don traveled to Bangkok, Thailand, for stem cell treatment on his heart. And, in fact, Don's life was probably extended to some degree because of his treatment in Bangkok.

I will never forget that moment when I was teaching my multicultural education course at the university and my cell phone rang with a strange ring tone. Usually my phone is on vibrate or turned off, but it was ringing. I looked down to see an unrecognizable number. I begged forgiveness from my students and answered the call, right in front of class. I heard, "Eh, dis Professor Awesome?" (That was Don's nickname for me. When we first met, I was in the habit of using the word "Awesome" in response, quite often, to his questions like, "How do I look?" Because of his vanity and my persistence in using the word, it became his nickname for me.)

He was actually calling me from his hospital bed in Bangkok to tell me he had talked to his stem cell team in Bangkok about using stem cells to treat autoimmune diseases. He said the doctors told him the research wasn't quite there yet, but not to give up. They believed that breaking into the world of stem cell treatment for autoimmune diseases was right around the corner.

That he called me from his hospital bed half a world away to tell me he had consulted his doctors on my behalf illustrated that our friendship was as important to him as it was to me. Don continued to push for a cure for my illnesses or at least to find more effective treatment. When he died, I began to lose hope for myself.

The psychiatrist I started seeing was a perfect match for me. There was no doubt he would be a starter on my team and I would continue to talk with him on a regular basis. I have enough experience with therapy through the years (and I've tried on many different shapes and sizes of therapy) to know when you find something or someone who just "fits," you don't let it go. My psychiatrist didn't just listen and ask thought-provoking questions, he also had two-way communication with me to provide a verbal outlet for talking through my ideas. Our conversations often reminded me of having coffee with a mentor; both parties asking questions and both parties adding to the knowledge base.

I continued seeing him up until I left for Turkey. Afterwards, as soon as I got the all clear from my stem cell doctor that I could leave my house for more than thirty minutes a day, I scheduled an appointment with my psychiatrist.

In general, things seemed good, in terms of no symptoms resurrecting themselves, for about a year post-transplant. In 2012, reality set in that I was actually going to live, and I realized my focus needed to shift to learning how to live instead of waiting to die. I had spent a lifetime waiting to die, and suddenly (well, maybe not so suddenly) the playing field had changed. I had outgrown my psychiatrist. The two-way communication I was used to having during each session turned into me being talking out loud with very little verbal or non-verbal response. In retrospect, I wonder if he realized the circumstances had changed so dramatically. Once my neuro-psychological testing was complete, and the detailed results were available, it was clear that continuing treatment with my long-time psychiatrist was not going to be time-effective, cost-effective, or even solution-effective.

How was I going to tell him I wouldn't be coming back? How could I explain to him that I appreciated the years of financial assistance he had gifted me when my bills were so high that I couldn't afford my counseling co-pay, that it was time for me to find a doctor who had more experience in different areas? I felt indebted to this doctor. He was someone who knew me better than I knew myself at times. He had helped me to move on again after losing my best friend. I knew I had no choice; I had to sit this player on the bench not just for my benefit, but for his, too.

I scheduled one last appointment with him. The first thing I did was share with him the results of the testing by my cognitive rehabilitation therapist and the plan we created to try and get my working life back on track. For the first time in months, he showed interest and joy in my own excitement. I told him I planned to do cognitive rehabilitation every week and felt like I needed to focus my time on that right now. He agreed with me.

I had been dreading that appointment. I was afraid I would disappoint him. What I found was a that I could employ a teaching tool I was taught long ago by my co-author when I was in high school: she told me that good teachers, when providing feedback to students or dealing with parents, always start with the positive and move into what needs improvement. Before our session was over, he asked me to call his office every now and again to let him know how I was doing. He told me I didn't need to schedule an appointment, just give a quick check in.

Making the hard choice to sit a player is never easy, especially when you genuinely like the person. But it has to be done. Remember, your team MUST change over time. Making even a simple change in your health care (changing medications, trying a new treatment plan) can ultimately decide who the starters will be on your team at any given time. And just because your lineup changes and starters become bench warmers, doesn't mean those bench warmers won't be needed at a later time.

Summary

I have no doubt that you need to make your own decisions about the members of your medical team (your defensive line) and which of these doctors will be the quarterback. If you are as lucky as I was, your offensive line (your *'ohana*) will step up and help you get through the toughest parts of your journey. When I think about my experience, it occurs to me that it has been a much more organic process than I anticipated when I thought about writing this book, which may mean that my experience is not something that you can replicate.

My best advice is, I think, to surround yourself with competent doctors who have your own best interests at heart. Go into your appointments with them armed with as much knowledge as you can come up with. Make sure they know that you would like to be a partner in the entire process of your health care and that you can be a competent partner. It should make a difference.

Additionally, be prepared for surprises, changes, disappointments along the line, but NEVER give up. You are your own best advocate; you are the expert on you. Make sure they recognize that.

Just Remember

- You must take responsibility to lead (coach) the team of doctors with whom you are working.

Make certain you are knowledgeable and well informed about your condition(s) in order to gain their respect.

- When you are dealing with multiple diagnoses and multiple doctors, it is critical that your doctors work as a team. Each one needs to know what the others are doing and how they can work together in your best interest.

- Don't be afraid to change doctors when health circumstances change.

- Pull together your support network (your *'ohana*) and let them do for you what you cannot do for yourself.

S.T.E.P.S. in Action: Teamwork

The easiest way to demonstrate Teamwork in Action is to share with you changes in my team as the stem cell transplant became a reality.

You know that old football play, the Quarterback Sneak? Well, Dr. Uramoto and I called it. We spent a lot of time looking for openings into the end zone for a stem cell transplant. To do that, Team Hawaii needed fresh players. Enter WorldMed Assist and Janet Kwan. Janet would be the equivalent of a special teams coach who came on board to introduce the new players in the fall of 2010.

Janet is a registered nurse (RN, BSN) who works for WorldMed Assist, one of the companies I found doing my Google search for medical tourism. So why did I decide to go with Janet and her company? Because she made me feel like I was the only patient she was working with. She made me feel important and valued. The Better Business Bureau had given WorldMed Assist an A+ rating, not that it mattered. What mattered more were the hospitals Janet worked with and their affiliations with US hospitals.

By December, 2010, Janet had connected me with Dr. Gülbaş and Dilek Inci, the patient advocate at Anadolu Medical Center near Istanbul, Turkey. Anadolu is joint commission approved and is partnered with Johns Hopkins Medicine. Joint commission approval is a very big deal. Ask any nurse what it means and they will talk for about thirty minutes nonstop sharing horror stories about joint commission visits. And then they will smile happily and say, "In the end we got it." And now I was developing two Super Bowl teams! Team Hawaii and Team Turkey.

It's not very often that your starting quarterback agrees to sit out one of the most important games for the team. However, in my case, we did not have any other options. You may remember me mentioning that Dr. Gülbaş had consulted with me and Dr. Uromoto in Honolulu. You might also wonder how that happened. Once Janet had made the connection between Dr. Gülbaş and me, I received an email from Dilek asking if I would agree to meet Dr. Gülbaş while he was in Hawaii. Wait, what?!?! Dr. Gülbaş is coming here? To Hawaii? Okay, yeah, that's a no brainer; of course I will meet him and even do one better. I will take him to meet Dr. Uramoto.

Fast forward to February, just two weeks before Liz and I were to leave for Turkey and the evening before this epic doctor's appointment, I had to call Dr. Gülbaş at his hotel. He was in Hawaii for an international conference on bone marrow/stem cell transplants. Wow! How cool was that? I was so nervous having to call him, just like the first time I ever called someone to go on a date. Sweaty palms nervous. Needless to say, the call was successful and Dr. Gülbaş didn't run away because I was flubbing up all my thoughts and words. The next morning, Liz and I picked him up in front of his hotel and off we went to meet Dr. Uramoto. (Some details of the meeting are described in Chapter 5.)

What I need to highlight here, under S.T.E.P.S in Action, is that Dr. Gülbaş would not have moved forward with my stem cell transplant had Dr. Uramoto failed to answer one very important question correctly. Dr. Gülbaş asked Dr. Uramoto, point blank, "Do you recommend Cristy as a candidate for a peripheral blood stem cell transplant?" Had Dr. Uramoto said "no" everything would have stopped right there because Dr. Gülbaş needed to hear her approval. You might think this is a strange question for him to ask at that point, since it appeared the transplant would soon be a done deal, but he had a very good reason. It is because many rheumatologists still do not support autologous stem cell transplant as a viable treatment plan for autoimmune disease. Looking back now, I wish I had recorded this meeting.

You will discover, if you research autoimmune disorders and diseases on the Internet, that major medical agencies in the US, such as the National Institutes of Health and the Mayo Clinic, make no mention of stem cell transplant as a treatment, so I was very fortunate to have found a rheumatologist who could see the promise of such treatment.

Dr. Gülbaş told Liz and me many times in the past three years that Dr. Uramoto is a very progressive-thinking doctor in her field and he has a lot of respect for her. With Dr. Uramoto's seal of approval, she handed the ball off to Dr. Gülbaş so he could run into the end zone to score the transplant.

From December 2010 through April 2011 Team Turkey was on the field with Dr. Gülbaş calling the plays, while Team Hawaii sat out as spectators. (See Figure 6.)

Team Turkey (until April 2011)	Transition Team (May 2011-March 2012)	Current Team
• Janet Kwan, WorldMed Assist • Dr. Zafer Gülbaş, Professor of Internal Medicine and Hematology and Quarterback • Dilek Inci, Patient Advocate, Anadolu Medical Center • Banu, Nurse Manager, Transplant Ward, Anadolu Medical Center • Nurses in Transplant Ward • Nurses in Oncology Ward • Microbiologist • Cardiologist	• Dr. Gülbaş • Dr. Uramoto, Rheumatologist and Quarterback • Dilek Inci • Dr. L General Practitioner	• Dr. Uramoto • Dr. L • Dr. Gülbaş • Dilek Inci • Gastroenterologist twice a year for monitoring • Dermatologist twice a year for monitoring • Occupational therapist • Neuropsychologist and psychiatrist transition to living and dealing with chemo brain

Figure 6: Changes in quarterback position and defensive lineup between December 2010 and the present.

Your team MUST change as your health changes. Since I have done this in Hawaii, as well as other states, and in Bangkok and Turkey, what I know to be absolute fact is that when I decided to coach my own team, transitions became smooth and usually involve lasting collaboration among all the players.

CHAPTER 4—STEP 3: EDUCATION

Education is the most powerful weapon you can use to change the world.
Nelson Mandela

Education is the third step in my process of being your own patient advocate. That doesn't mean it is third in relevance. Actually, all five steps work together simultaneously in concert with one another. (Well, actually, it is the third step because it gives me the vowel I need to make S.T.E.P.S. an acronym.) I am going to divide this chapter into three areas. The first is education as it relates to the patient, or me and you. Second, I will talk about education and your medical team. And third, I want to explore the role of education in the lives of your offensive line (spouses/partners, family, friends, and colleagues who are supporting you on your journey).

The most important aspect in terms of education is that you need to become an expert on you. You may get tired of hearing this, but this is the biggest, most important aspect of becoming your own patient advocate.

Education and the Patient

Has anyone ever told you, when you aren't feeling well or have an injury, to avoid searching the Internet for information? Do they remind you that too many Internet sites are unreliable? Or have they said that you should at least be wary of those people (frequently patients) or sites (frequently blogs) that are one-sided, being one person's point of view without expert analysis? And have you maybe wondered, as I often do, why people really feel the need to tell you this?

Reality for those of us dealing with a health care crisis is that if we are investigating the disease(s) online or searching for available treatments, then we are smart enough to determine what is valuable information versus what is not. I say this because I believe I am a relatively smart person and capable of reading all kinds of material and discerning what is relevant to me and my condition(s). So my advice? Learn as much as you can. Read the good, happy success stories and celebrate the storyteller's good fortune. Read the horror stories; they will help you recognize red flags and things to watch out for. Read academic papers written by experts; you may not understand everything in such documents, but you can glean a great deal of helpful information from them. Give yourself a broad range of knowledge-based tools so you can intellectually survive the inevitable barrage of medical terminology related to diagnoses and treatment options. For instance, by the time I arrived in Turkey I knew the peripheral stem cell transplant process inside and out, and, because of that, nothing—I mean nothing— came as a surprise. When Dr. Gülbaş asked to meet with my partner and me the morning after we arrived, he was impressed with how much knowledge we had brought with us. It wasn't long before he said, "Okay, we can start the paperwork and you can be admitted this afternoon to start chemotherapy." I had no hesitation in saying, "Let's roll." Neither Liz nor I needed to have him explain everything in detail, and he appreciated that we had done our homework.

As a patient, you give yourself super powers by becoming educated on your own case. This doesn't mean telling your well-educated quarterback or members of your defensive line what to do. It DOES mean that you can engage in two-way conversation about relevant data related to diagnosis and treatment. Education is only as powerful as you let it be. And for me, I found that the more educated

I was, the more likely I would finally succeed in getting my stem cell transplant. I literally had to work against the FDA and insurance companies to get what I needed. And I guess if I had really educated myself on patient rights as they relate to my health coverage, I might have spent time legally appealing to my insurance company's denial of coverage. This would have been a huge waste of time, and I did not have time to spare. My health had deteriorated to a point where I could spend my energy on finding treatment or spend it with an attorney (in which case I may not have been alive to see results of the appeal).

The first time I needed to be educated in my own healthcare began when I was trying to figure out if I had Chiari malformation (2000). I had essentially self-diagnosed the problem by tracking my symptoms and studying possible disorders or diseases related to those symptoms. A friend of mine had undergone surgery for Chiari malformation, and she referred me to her neurosurgeon at Johns Hopkins Hospital in Baltimore. I called this doctor and was told I could get an appointment but I would need to bring the results of an MRI with me when I came. But since I was operating from a self-diagnosis, I had not yet had an MRI, and finding someone to write the orders for one was going to be tricky, or so I thought.

I had stopped seeing my GP (you know, the one who had told me I was a hypochondriac) and was now seeing a doctor at University of Maryland (UM) Medical Center. I wasn't quite sure if the doctor at UM would be willing to write MRI orders since the bulk of his work didn't involve this kind of diagnostic testing. I started looking for a neurologist, but I found the wait would be extremely long to get in, and before they would consider ordering an MRI they would first require another line of diagnostic testing. It was discouraging.

By now, though, I was absolutely certain I had Chiari malformation, Type I. I had done a lot of research online, mostly looking at medical journals, and I had very little doubt this was one of the health issues I was dealing with. It all added up and made sense. Specifically, I have a very small head (and I still wear children's-sized ball caps); headaches had been a problem for as long as I can remember. I had first noticed something unusual about my headaches when I had to do gymnastics in gym class. If I did one somersault, it inevitably led to a major migraine; finally, there was the injury I had sustained my sophomore year in college, which ended my soccer career. I found that Chiari malformation Type I, although congenital, is often triggered by trauma later in life.

I decided to take a chance and make an appointment with the doctor my friend had recommended and explain to him what I had found. Lo and behold, he listened to me— he actually listened to me and ordered the MRI. He told me he was impressed with the information I had brought in and had no problem ordering the MRI to either confirm or rule out Chiari malformation. I suspect if I had gone to see him without the knowledge I had, he probably would have put me through a long series of diagnostic tests prior to ordering the MRI. I think it's a bit rare for a doctor to order an MRI as a result of a conversation with a patient on her first visit.

With the MRI scheduled, I decided I wanted to know how doctors determine if Chiari malformation is present. What would the MRI show? As noted in the previous chapter, Chiari malformation occurs when the bottom part of the cerebellum—the tonsils—descend into the upper spinal canal and interfere with the flow of cerebral spinal fluid. I learned all about cerebral tonsils and how far they needed to be descended for a diagnosis. I knew that the MRI would show how far mine had descended.

I even found a series of diagrams demonstrating how a neurosurgeon reads the MRI and measures the displacement of the cerebellar tonsils. I went in for my MRI, which, of course, was in the day when they shoved you into a very narrow capsule, an unbearably noisy capsule, with only earplugs to (ineffectively) deaden the sound. Nowadays, you get television, radio, or at least music to help distract you from the noise and the close quarters in the machine. When they pulled me out of the MRI machine, I asked the technician if I could see my scans. He agreed and let me come into the office where the images were on the computer. I asked him to enlarge one of the slides and pulled a plastic ruler from my pocket. I pointed to the screen and said these are my cerebellar tonsils and then I measured them, finding a seven millimeter displacement. I told the technician that I definitely had Chiari malformation. He was speechless at first and then he laughed and said yes, you're right, but I'm not supposed to tell the patient what the scan shows. I told him he didn't tell me anything; I only asked him to see my scan. It was a funny moment for sure, and each subsequent time I would go for a follow-up MRI, I tried to go when he was working just because he was so fascinated by the disease and treatment and by my brains, which seemed to be too big for my head.

I should mention that diagnosis for Chiari malformation is improving as technology is allowing doctors to do even more specific testing to determine extent of the cranial fluid obstruction.

Learning as much as you can about your illness is important to being the best coach you can be, not because you want to dictate to your doctors what they should be doing, but because you deserve to know as much as you can about your own body and to understand everything the doctor tells you. Again, some people will tell you to stay away from websites, social media outlets, or blogs where people are telling their stories. I disagree, look at everything you can find and sort it out. Some sites will be valuable, others may be poorly documented and unreliable, but you should be able to sift through it to find nuggets of wisdom.

My health care journey has been interesting in terms of the Internet and social media. When I first started dealing with multiple, non-specific, strange symptoms, I didn't have Internet at home and the one at the school where I worked was on a dial-up connection. You remember those days? No Google, no Yahoo, just an Internet link from my school to the local public library system. Occasionally, I would spend my planning period searching for books about my symptoms, but it wasn't until the mid-90s that I had easy access to the 'net that I really began to find the resources I needed.

By 1998, I was beginning to see more medical resources available and was able to educate myself about Chiari malformation. During this time, though, I listened to the so-called experts who advised me to stay away from sites that focused just on one patient's experiences. I believed my doctors when they said that people who post their medical stories on the Internet were just those with rare examples of complications or tragic endings. Eventually, though, my curiosity got the best of me and I ventured into those sites.

What I found, once I started reading these sites, is that there were patients like me and patients not like me. But regardless of our exact situations, I found people who could relate to certain things I was experiencing. For example, much later, when I returned home after my transplant in 2011, I started getting vicious headaches and my legs ached all the time. It scared me and I wondered if the stem cell transplant had been for naught; I posted a question about these symptoms on a blog for stem cell transplant survivors, who could easily identify with what I was describing. Several people responded, and I found that both symptoms could be caused by the anti-bacterial drug, Bactrim, one of the medications I was taking post-transplant because infections could be deadly. Although I had to stay on that particular medication, the dosage was reduced to every other day and the symptoms were relieved. I not only want to hear from patients who can relate to me in ways no one else can, I need to hear from them. No matter how many transplants a doctor performs, unless they have gone through it themselves, pain can be misunderstood.

One of my medical heroes is a guy I first met via Twitter who lives in the United Kingdom. When I met Michael

Seres in person in the summer of 2013, I discovered we were kindred spirits regarding the role of social media in connecting us to others who, like us, have navigated or are now navigating the medical maze and the stem cell transplant process. Michael said something that has stuck with me ever since. He said, "If I am feeling something in my body that doesn't seem right or is a new symptom for me, I take comfort in knowing I can get online and reach out to others who can relate. They matter."

Educating myself about the research, about other patients, and about treatment options was and is key to my survival. Although I am almost three years post-transplant, I still need to keep learning all that I can about life after stem cell transplant. Long-term data is still relatively slim and so with each day I live, I enter new territory as a survivor. As most cancer survivors will tell you, the thought that the disease has returned is always in the back of your mind. I continue to be a student in all things autoimmune and stem cell transplant so that as my recovery continues I am prepared for any valley or peak.

Education and Your Medical Team

I am here to tell you my medical team is the best. Okay, the best team for me. You need your medical team to be the best team for you. This requires some mutual respect and mutual learning. Sometimes the patient is the one who has to be the teacher, or to at least start the lesson. This only works, though, if the team demonstrates mutual respect to and for each other.

Once upon a time I had a chance to see a local doctor (in Hawaii) about the possibility of a stem cell transplant. His reputation had preceded him and I was scared to visit him by myself. I knew he was well respected in his specialization and I knew his success rate, but I had learned from others that his bedside manner was seriously lacking. I needed to see this doctor. If I were going to have a chance to have a stem cell transplant in my home state, I needed to work with and through this doctor. I decided to ask my quarterback (my rheumatologist) to go with me to my consultation. I told her that I would pay for a regular office visit and I would work around any time and date that was convenient for her. To this day I'm not sure if she ever billed me, but I know for a fact that by saying I would pay for an office visit, I was able to show her that I valued her input, her time and her expertise. But beyond that, the fact that she agreed to join me for this consultation showed that she also respected me as a knowledgeable patient, someone she was willing to go an extra mile for to help find treatment.

Before we went for the stem cell consultation, my rheumatologist and I had four and half years' worth of research studies and statistics on the impact of SCT on scleroderma patients, open studies available in the United States, open studies happening in Hawaii, and pounds of information from my medical file (I literally mean pounds). Together, my rheumatologist and I had been educating ourselves on every treatment option available for scleroderma patients. We were as prepared as we were going to be for this consultation.

The consultation was conducted in the other doctor's office and included my rheumatologist, my partner, Liz, and me. It went surprisingly well as the doctor about whom I had heard horror stories turned out to be nice, attentive, and very interested in my case. We provided solid information about scleroderma, vasculitis, and ankylosing spondylitis with SCT as a treatment option, which apparently made him comfortable enough to say I was a great candidate for a stem cell transplant. He said he would present my case to his medical team. Before we left, we explained to him that my health insurance had denied coverage, but that we would have the cash available up front if he agreed to do the transplant. (We were confident our fund-raising efforts would provide for the cost.) He told us we would hear from his office within a week with a decision.

When we left the doctor's office, my rheumatologist, Liz and I all felt like we had struck gold. We all honestly believed he would accept my case.

Almost two weeks later I received a call from the doctor's receptionist setting an appointment for me to come back and meet with him. Again, we felt even more positive because, if it was going to be bad news, he wouldn't waste his office time. Right? Uh, yeah, no. He wanted that appointment and he even charged me for it. Liz and I sat in his waiting room for an hour. When we were finally taken back to an examination room, we waited another twenty-five minutes. Then the doctor came in and with no hello, how are ya, no courtesies at all, he proceeded to tell us he had discussed my case with his colleagues and they decided they wouldn't take my case. Looking back on it I was shocked, but not totally caught off guard—I had become so used to disappointment. The prospect of the procedure had really been too good to be true. My partner, though, was astonished. Liz asked him what made him go from being so positive and saying I was great candidate to turning us down flat? Eventually he fessed up: if they accepted cash for the transplant they would lose future insurance incentives. Translation? Kickbacks.

The moral of this fairy tale, you ask? There are multiple morals. On the one hand, it illustrates the difficulty that patients in my situation find themselves. Had I been able to get the SCT in my home state of Hawaii, our fund-raising efforts would have easily covered the cost. But because I had to leave the country and travel half way around the world, the cost effectively doubled. Without the fund-raising efforts of my *'ohana*, this doctor's refusal of treatment could have been a death sentence. Furthermore, it shows an example of a doctor who believes medically, through his own research and education, that a patient should receive a treatment protocol, but whose hands are tied in spite of facts, the data, case studies, and other research, a doctor who cannot advocate for a life-saving procedure or treatment that conflicts with the rules of the almighty Health Insurance Company or the FDA. Oh, and it also illustrates how a doctor acts toward a patient when another medical doctor is in the room versus how he acts when it's just the doctor and the patient.

Finally, this is a great example of positive communication, mutual learning, and mutual respect between a doctor (my rheumatologist) and a patient (me). It shows the dedication of an amazing doctor to her patient by her willingness to investigate all possibilities and walk the journey with the patient.

I mentioned in the previous chapter how I developed my relationship with my quarterback in terms of using email so appointment time wasn't wasted. Most of the research we both discovered on treatments and transplants for patients like me, we shared via email. The greatest thing about my relationship with my quarterback was if I emailed her information on a study and she felt I would benefit from it, she would reach out to make contact with any doctor necessary. This included doctors in Bangkok and Turkey. The comfort of email for me as a patient was that I could send an email any time day or night and know she would read it when she had time. I knew I wouldn't disturb her work schedule or personal time by having her paged. Respect is needed for developing your team; it is also needed when the doctor and patient are learning new things together.

Education and Your Offensive Line

Have you ever tried to explain an algebraic equation to a four-year-old? No? Me neither, but I would imagine it would be something similar to explaining whole-body pain to someone who has never been in a hospital except to give birth or to visit others who are sick. If you're lucky, that person may have had an experience where they, also, have experienced pain, localized or total body, which may have been the result of injury or accident. Such experiences might give them a bit of perspective on what you are describing.

But, to be blunt here, unless the person you are talking to has dealt with the exact same disease, injury, or symptom exactly the same as you, then guess what, they ain't gonna get it. As hard as this concept is for the patient (you) to understand, it is even harder for the person listening to you to understand that they can't possibly get it. This is especially true in regards to autoimmune diseases, which are not easily understood and which are often manifested in whole-body pain. This can lead to a breakdown in communication and, even worse, in relationships. Helping your offensive line to empathize with you is more important than having them completely understand you. I do know that this can be minimized when education plays a part in your relationships with your offensive line. This means finding a way to share with those closest to you what you have been learning and allowing them to share with you what they may have been discovering during their own research.

The *One of Our Own Fund* website did the most to help my 'ohana become knowledgeable about my illnesses and my progress toward treatment. We posted detailed descriptions of the symptoms I was experiencing, explanations and links to more detailed explanations of the autoimmune disorders I was suffering from, and kept a running commentary on my treatment options and our preparation for the stem cell transplant.

Liz's blog, *From Here to Istanbul*, provided an eyewitness account of the procedures I underwent in Turkey. I suspect my 'ohana knows more today about autoimmune diseases and stem cell transplants than the average person.

Your Inner Circle: Within your offensive line, there are probably a number of people who could be considered your "inner circle." These are the folks who know as much as they possibly can about you, and you them, without living under the same roof or being intimately involved.

These are the people who rally others to support and continue to support you on the journey.

My inner circle has changed over time as my team changed over time. I mentioned in the previous chapter that your offensive line will change, sometimes by choice, although sometimes it's beyond anyone's control. Moving to Hawaii changed my inner circle. My inner circle would continue to change even more once it was known that Liz was my chosen life partner (details for another time, I suppose). And changes have occurred over and through time, there are some that are still at the core and always will be. I wouldn't be sitting here writing this story without my inner circle and most importantly those who chose to be part of the *One of Our Own Fund* team.

Helping to educate my inner circle was easy. This was because they wanted to understand how they could help me. As Liz and I would discover new information, we would often share with others in the inner circle via email, then through the original *One of Our Own Fund* website which went online in early 2010, and finally through the blog, From Here to Istanbul, when Liz and I traveled to Turkey (2011) for the transplant. Even after the transplant, updates on the website continued to spread the news about my recovery.

An educated inner circle oftentimes offers support to you in ways you never knew would or could exist. This is how the *One of Our Own Fund* team started and began to raise funds for my transplant—and this was even before we knew I would have to leave the country for it. Through the website, our webmaster (Sharon, who is also my co-author) introduced me to the world by telling my story and describing the medical issues I faced. She posted updates on my condition and the progress of my diseases and treatments. She put up a PayPal link and sent out regular emails soliciting donations to meet my medical expenses, which were building dangerously high. It was important to post updates regularly and to reach out to additional people, taking my story beyond what I considered my inner circle. The website became an extremely important means of educating a large number of people.

Most importantly, when Liz and I were exhausted and overwhelmed by the illnesses, our inner circle would band together to provide the encouragement we would need to persevere (which I will discuss in the next chapter).

Your inner circle, like mine, also includes family members who may not be with you day in and day out, but are supporting you through prayer and love. My entire family still lives on the East Coast, with the exception of my stepbrother and his family who are located halfway between me and the East Coast. This geographical separation made it difficult sometimes when I needed them to understand my daily health troubles. Because they didn't see me from day to day, it was impossible to see how I was wearing down from the pain I was in. They knew I was continuing to work, so I imagine some of them wondered just how sick I really was. It's hard to explain the drive to function normally in a fog of pain and discomfort, knowing all the while that your own body is trying to kill you. I had to keep working; otherwise, I might have given in to the despair and hopelessness that shadowed me every single day. The best I could do was try to educate them about these terrible diseases by sharing as much detail as I could about what I was feeling. Perhaps one of the most important educational tools was Liz's blog, From Here to Istanbul, which she wrote after we left for the transplant. Her blog helped them learn even more about the transplant procedure and, probably most importantly, the progress I began to make almost immediately.

Acquaintances and Colleagues: Also in your offensive line are those acquaintances and colleagues who may only know you from work or from other activities. They are not necessarily your intimate friends, and they may not know everything that has been going on with you medically. In a perfect world, all people we meet would be educated enough to know everything we know and understand about our illness. Or at least know as much as our inner circle.

But this is not a perfect world, and we always have people who think they know more than we ever could about the medical journey we are walking. I come back to the notion that my education, and yours, is critical. It is vital for you to learn as much as you can so that no matter what comments you hear from others, you know without a doubt that what you are doing is the right thing. For some people in this category, providing them with knowledge is well received and interpreted, and they take an interest in supporting and helping you. Others? They will either get it or not; they will look up some things on WebMD, consider themselves experts, and doubt your knowledge of your own condition. These are the same people who will question your veracity because you continue to work and meet your day-to-day obligations, because, of course, there's no way you could do that if you were really sick. Nothing you say will change their perceptions. Again, trust yourself, your closest allies, and your doctors and stay the course, which is sometimes difficult. I'll explore that more fully in the next chapter.

Education and Your Care Giver

I could have made this section a part of the previous one, since my care giver is an important part of my offensive line, but I think she deserves a heading of her own. I should begin by clarifying what I mean by "care giver," that, for this book, I mean the person who is walking most closely with you on your journey. I need to distinguish between the single word, "caregiver" and my use of two words: "care giver." A caregiver is quite often a professional who is hired to provide direct care to a sick person. A care giver is the person who cares about you the most, not necessarily the person who cares for you when you are bedridden or just too sick to do anything for yourself.

Your care giver is likely your spouse, partner, parent, sibling, child, or anyone else who is the one who becomes your "go to" person. For a very long time in my health care journey, I did things alone. There was no one walking the journey with me. Not that this is a bad thing, but if your health continues to deteriorate, chances are pretty good you will need to turn to someone to help get you through treatment, doctor visits, hospital visits, and so forth. For each of us our care giver may be defined differently, but regardless of other definitions, for you, this is the person who is there for you through it all.

After my move to Hawaii and I was diagnosed with cancer (2005), I was still pretty much flying solo. But even then, I had my dear friend, Don Ho, nearby and another friend from Maryland who came to stay with me for the first week after I returned home from surgery. Eventually, though, after I could no longer mask the deterioration of my health, I was blessed to find Liz. I hope our experience of learning together and working together to find treatment can help you and your care giver as you travel on your own journey.

When I first met Liz we spent hours meeting for coffee and talking about all kinds of things, but actually not much about my health problems. I was initially reluctant to tell her that I might be dying. One day I dropped four words on her that had her scrambling for a computer and Google. I said, "scleroderma, vasculitis, ankylosing spondylitis." The very instant I spoke these four words, I followed it with "chronic, progressive, and deadly." From that moment on, I knew she would travel this road with me. Liz and I worked together to learn as much as we could. She was as committed to learning as I was.

One of the greatest things about Liz was that she never grew tired of learning about my diseases. She didn't burn out as some others had during my journey. Liz had a way of sharing new things she had read or found online that added to our knowledge base; she never talked down to me or implied that I had not done as much research as I should have. Liz willingly agreed to walk my journey with me, even knowing death was coming for me sooner rather than later. One of the ways were able to keep our conversations positive, without upsetting each other, was to share links, articles, statistics, research studies, and doctor appointments with one another. Even though there were times early on after I met Liz that I still wanted to fly solo on doctor's visits, she insisted that she go. And eventually it felt strange if she wasn't there.

The lesson here is that it is just as important to educate your care giver as it is yourself. Don't try to protect your care giver from knowledge of your illnesses. Don't keep secrets. It helps if both of you are willing to learn together. By the time we arrived in Turkey and the chemotherapy, which is preliminary to the stem cell transplant, had started, Liz knew exactly what to expect and that if any situation arose, she could speak for me. And not just speak for me out of an emotional context, but also as an educated voice that understood exactly what was necessary according to what we learned and what we knew to be grounded in best practice.

Summary

NBC's *The More You Know Campaign*, which has been broadcast on the network since 1989, is one of my favorite ideas for helping to educate the public about important societal issues. Their powerful public service announcements are short sound bites, usually twenty seconds or less, promoting positive action or behavior that makes you think about something and potentially act on it. I wish I could develop sound bites like these about all three of my autoimmune diseases, the major symptoms, and the treatments I've endured. I would download them all to my smart phone or tablet and whenever I needed to inform someone about my medical history, I could whip it out and hit play. Wouldn't it be cool to have Mr. Rogers do a twenty-second blurb on chemotherapy? Maybe that will be my next venture. For now, though, it is important to remember that the more you know about you, the stronger you become. Your mind is just as important in your medical journey as your body.

And before I leave this chapter I would like to say a word to all the WebMD "experts": Before you impart your new found expert knowledge on a patient who is suffering with chronic or terminal illness, try asking her first what she already knows through her own research. You may be surprised by how much more the patient knows than you, along with how many times she may have tried to get into an FDA-sanctioned research trial in the United States in the previous five years before you Googled the disease. I don't want to imply that I am an expert, but my guess is that I am more informed about my diseases than the person who surfed the web and found WebMD.

Sometimes the problem is that my explanations come off like a Reader's Digest condensed version. Remember that time you were in a fender bender and you needed to recount all of the details to the cop, to the insurance company, to the auto shop, to your significant other, to your boss, to your friends? By the time you hit the third or fourth retelling you probably were exhausted by all the details and shortened the story to include basics necessary to inform the person(s) you were telling. This is the same for a patient struggling with a major disease. We try our best to keep everyone informed, but sometimes the best we can do is give the condensed version, which might just fall short for some people.

Just Remember

- Research, research, research! The Internet is your friend, but use it wisely.

- Use the information your body is giving you (sensibility) to investigate symptoms and treatment.

- Share information with your doctors in a collaborative way; let them know you are doing everything you can to help them get to diagnoses and treatments.

- Share information with your support network (your *'ohana*) so they know and understand the best ways to help you.

- Don't keep secrets about your condition from the people who mean the most to you. Let them walk with you on your journey.

S.T.E.P.S. in Action: Education

Pre-Transplant

As I mentioned before, I knew things weren't right with my body after my hysterectomy and, yes, I was right in terms of needing to follow up with Meckel's Diverticulum and the cancerous growth in the small intestine. Even with those issues taken care of, I still didn't feel like my old self. (I know my old self wasn't normal by a long stretch, but my old self was different; at least it was manageable.)

Then something else—something totally new and alarming—hit me out of nowhere; the strangest thing happened while I was swimming in the ocean. My face and lips swelled up like I was having a "Nutty Professor" moment. ("The Nutty Professor" was an Eddie Murphy movie in which he played a morbidly obese university professor.) My lips were so swollen it felt like they were going to rip open. They burned and hurt. My forehead was two times its normal size. It was weird, but also extremely frightening.

After several hours, the swelling and pain subsided, but I made an appointment with my general practitioner for as soon as possible. This doctor's visit sent me off on a new path to educate myself about what the heck happened to my face. My GP sent me to an immunologist, who sent me to a dermatologist, who finally sent me to a rheumatologist. And so my defensive line was born.

I learned from the immunologist, after a lot of allergy testing, that my biggest and most severe allergies were to dogs and cats. That wasn't new information for me, since I had a cat at the time and had been on daily allergy medication to head off symptoms. Yet, she found no reasonable explanation for the swelling of my lips. The dermatologist was unable to recreate the hives-like reaction using ice, as both he and the immunologist thought maybe I had a reaction typical to cold uticaria (hives). But the dermatologist, the same doctor who would eventually tell me I needed to have a quarterback and I needed to be the coach, had the idea that maybe something was going on in my body that could be associated with an autoimmune disease.

Together, the dermatologist and immunologist ordered blood panels and other various diagnostic tests. Yet we still didn't find anything definitive. I had some topical ointment from the dermatologist to use on my lips and face if swelling occurred again. The immunologist had prescribed numerous allergy medications. Still every time I went swimming, my lips and face would swell. So eventually I was given the dreaded, cure-all steroid medication, prednisone. Yes, it worked, but I refused to accept a non-definitive answer to the question of why I returned to shore looking like the nutty professor when I went swimming.

And then the weird lip swelling reaction happened again. But this time it was when I was eating chicken wings. Back to the immunologist I went and we looked again at all of the food allergies she tested me for initially. Still no link to be found. For me, the only thing I could think of was that both the wings, covered in Old Bay seasoning, and the ocean contain salt. After more prednisone and a careful review of my records, my immunologist scheduled me to consult with Dr. Uramoto, a rheumatologist, because she had a hunch that my issues were autoimmune related. Before I left her office, my immunologist gave me a friendly warning (probably because she knew I could be quite the persistent patient) that whatever was going on with my body was not definitively presenting itself. It is still evolving and common autoimmune diagnostic testing isn't giving us answers yet.

One week later I walked into Dr. Uramoto's office. And together we would learn to love learning as much as we could about evolving mixed connective tissue disease, clinical trials, and treatments.

For the first several months with Dr. Uramoto, every test she ordered came back with a resounding, "Nope, it's not.... " (You can fill in the blank with lupus, rheumatoid arthritis, multiple sclerosis). But in late 2006, Dr. Uramoto ordered a blood panel to test for the presence of HLA B27. (Human Leukocyte Antigens, which signal the presence of a protein in the surface of white blood cells, is found in patients with ankylosing spondylitis.) On my follow-up visit, Dr. Uramoto could finally say, "Yes, you tested positive for HLA B27, which means some of your symptoms are linked to ankylosing spondylitis."

I don't think I need to tell you how fast I Googled ankylosing spondylitis, but it was fast. I felt some relief because I could definitely pin the symptoms on a disease with a name. Then I started to search for cures, and that was when I first came to understand what a chronic, progressive disease is. Sure, AS probably wasn't going to kill me by itself, but it certainly would change my life and have me looking at eventually filing for disability.

In the meantime, I was still suffering with a whole other set of odd symptoms. I had all these little red spots showing up all along my veins; I had difficulty swallowing and keeping food down; and these crazy, big hive-like, blue and green bumps and streaks that traveled down both arms and legs. It didn't take Dr. Uramoto long to diagnose CREST syndrome: the tiny little red spots were telangiectasia, my swallowing issues were tied to esophageal dysmotility, and I had severe Raynaud's Syndrome caused by any temperature change inside or outside.

At this point in my medical journey I was seeing Dr. Uramoto once a month and she was able to make some diagnoses based on inclusion criteria versus definitive diagnostic tests. (Inclusion criteria are the standards by which a patient might be included in a clinical trial.) But even with the diagnoses, the best she could do for me was to prescribe medications to alleviate symptoms and try to slow down the progression of the diseases.

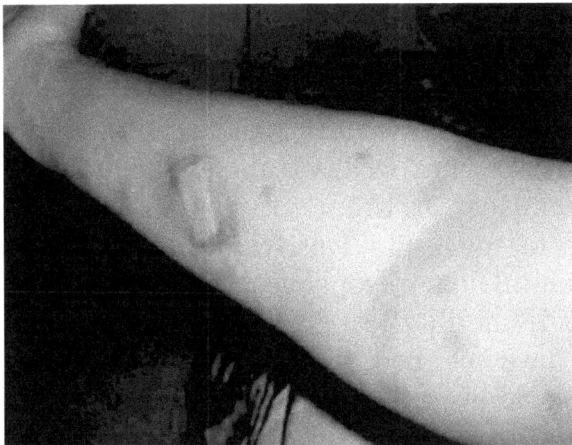

Vasculitis symptoms: painful bumps along the paths of blood vessels.

And the thing was, we still couldn't figure out why I was having these blue and green bumps appear. They were very painful, not itchy at all. There were times they felt like giant bruises. I had one on my lower shin that when touched was as painful as a broken bone. Often I would start out at Dr. Uramoto's office then head over to the dermatologist's office so he could do a biopsy. The second biopsy from my forearm gave us the vasculitis diagnosis.

My defensive line and I felt some relief at finally having a name, but like the other two diagnoses (ankylosing spondylitis and CREST Syndrome), the vasculitis was still evolving. Every time a new bump would appear in a new area or looked somewhat different, I had a biopsy. I had biopsies of these bumps that were so deep you could see bone. I had biopsies from my shins, back, shoulder, inner arms, ankle, and even at the base of my skull. That one was so deep and wide, even the nurse was surprised. Some biopsies came back inconclusive, so the dermatologist would go back in deeper and bigger. I got so used to it, I could have the biopsy done in the morning and then head right over to the university to teach.

Now that we had three names for three diseases, the really interesting part came into play. Knowing there was no cure for any of them, my best hope was to find the right combination of medicines that would ease the symptoms and stop the progression. Dr. Uramoto and I decided it would be a good idea for me to visit the Mayo Clinic in order to verify what we knew and determine the next best steps. I spent five full days at Mayo in 2007 and came away with even more respect for Dr. Uramoto. She definitely knows her specialty, and she is truly at the forefront of her profession. Mayo confirmed what we already knew, and I came home knowing that Dr. Uramoto and I were doing all of the right things for my health. I also came home with the definitive information on my esophageal dysmotility since Mayo ordered a dysmotility test. It is, by far, the worst diagnostic test I have ever had. I would do a colonoscopy standing on my head every week before I would do that test willingly again.

So let me paint you the picture. I got called into the exam room and was told to take a seat. The tech placed a pile of, like at least ten, bath towels across my lap and left them there. He then told me what was about to happen. He held up a very, very long tube that had a sensor/camera thingy in it, and said he was going to put it up my nose and down my throat into my stomach. Yeah, no response from me, just super huge eyes looking at him and that very, very long tube. Then he pointed out that the process causes a lot of people to gag, but if I just remember to breathe I won't gag. (Yeah, right.)

He said that once the tube was placed, he would give me some water, and when he told me to, I should take a sip and swallow only once. Any more than once, we'd have to do it again. After the water swallowing test, he said he'd give me a cracker and told me pretty much the same thing. I was to take a bite of the cracker and chew it for as long as he told me to, and then swallow only once. If I swallowed more than once, the swallow wouldn't count and we would have to do it over. Yeah, still no response from me, just shaking my head and feeling nauseous already.

Now that I knew the rules of this sadistic game, he moved toward me with the tube in his hand. With my eyes on the end of that tube, I asked him what the towels were for on my lap and he said just in case we need them. Then he was coming at me for real. He told me that if he had to stop pushing the tube down, he would have to pull it out and start over. So, in with the tube. I tried really hard to breathe and not gag, but I am here to tell you that having a tube shoved up your nose and down into your stomach is not an easy thing, unless maybe you are sedated. I can also tell you, for a fact, it is possible to not only gag when you are breathing but also to throw up. And then I knew why there were so many towels. As I puked on each one, he threw it to the floor and voilà, there was a clean one ready.

I made it through the test and learned that sixty percent of the time my esophagus did not work, leaving me unable to swallow both liquids and solids. Armed with that bit of knowledge, I left the lab feeling grateful for learning something important, but I couldn't help but wonder why anyone would ever want to do that job.

Upon my return to Hawaii, I started the long health care journey of trying different medications to keep my diseases at bay. But I also knew, as did my defensive line, that at the rate things were progressing, it would be just a matter of time before I wouldn't be able to teach anymore. I did not want that to happen and after a year of scouring the Internet, I became convinced that a stem cell transplant was the only treatment that might cure me (or not), but it could definitely put me into remission. A stem cell transplant, with my own stem cells, would allow me to keep teaching.

Post-Transplant

Even now that I am close to being three years post-transplant, I'm still learning things every day about stem cell transplants and long-term effects. Some of the effects I am experiencing now are not so good, like my issues with "chemo-brain." How do you deal with becoming ADHD (Attention Deficit Hyperactivity Disorder) in your forties? However, as each year passes more research is coming out in terms of the positive effects of SCT on autoimmune patients. A lot of this data is coming from Europe, but in actuality it doesn't matter as long as I can apply it to me.

Part of my continuing education has been through social media (Facebook and Twitter). Through both forums I found some interesting connections. In April, 2013, Liz and I attended a conference in Los Angeles just for stem cell and bone marrow transplant survivors and caregivers. I learned about this conference from Blood and Marrow Transplant Information Network, which I found via Facebook. The conference was interesting and gave Liz and me a lot to be so grateful for. We knew, without a doubt, we had made the right choice to go to Turkey for my transplant. The conference confirmed it for us. Had I waited much longer for a transplant, I'm sure I wouldn't be celebrating my forty-third birthday this year. I also learned about long-term effects of intense chemotherapy on lung function and realized that I would need to continue to have pulmonary function tests each year. While my lung function is somewhat diminished, it could get worse over time from the powerful chemotherapy I had prior to the transplant. I have to say, also, that finding other people who have gone through the transplant process is comforting. Not because we ALL still struggle with fatigue, but because they just "get it." I was shocked to find that many people do not return to work full time and end up on disability, so I count my blessings.

The most significant thing I took away from the conference was the concept of neuro-psychological testing. Shortly after I returned home, I had my neuro-psychological testing done. Since then I have been going every week for cognitive rehabilitation. I'm still not sure how it will all turn out, but through this process I am learning how to live; adapt to my new "normal."

Chapter 5—Step 4:
Perseverance and Patience

Patience and perseverance have a magical effect before which difficulties disappear and obstacles vanish.
John Quincy Adams

When I first identified my *5 S.T.E.P.S.* process, I only included patience for the "P" step. Sharon, my co-author, suggested we add perseverance as well. These two concepts work very closely together so I should probably revise the "P" to P². But when we tried it on the cover, it just looked odd. When you spend a lifetime trying to be patient, and you are finally able to get the treatment (or the outcome) you have been searching for, then it seems fitting to acknowledge that you have been persevering all along. But really, what exactly does that mean?

As with other steps in the process, I will define each of these terms so their definitions are consistent throughout for you and for me. Perseverance is steadfastness in doing something despite difficulty and delay in achieving success. Patience is the capacity to accept or tolerate delay, trouble, or suffering without getting angry or upset.

Perseverance

There are those events in our lives, and they happen to all of us, (not just to those people who can use hardship to "one up you in conversation"), that we decide to either overcome or succumb. In other aspects of this book I shared pretty clear-cut examples of each step. My perseverance is something I learned early in life.

I think I said before that I grew up as a tomboy and I idolized my dad; I wanted to do the best I could when I played sports so I could make him proud. My mom instilled in me from the beginning that no matter what you do, do it, and do it well. There are no excuses. Just do it. (Yes, she could have done marketing for Nike.)

If you take that scenario and you add in the fact that I had experienced pain for as far back as I could remember, the idea of succumbing to the pain/health issues was not an option.

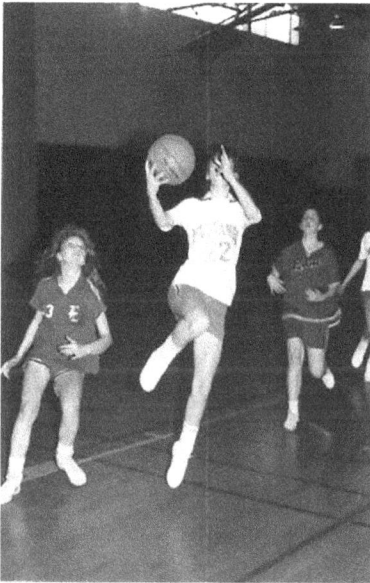

Cristy playing basketball at C. Milton Wright High School

One winter afternoon in 1989, when I was a senior in high school, I had basketball practice scheduled for 5:00 p.m. I had gone home from school and lay down only to wake up a bit later with pains in my chest. It was a different kind of pain, not the normal indigestion associated with what I would years later come to know as esophageal dysmotility, but a sharp pain followed by a dull throbbing. My mom was getting ready to go to work (she was on call for the operating room) and when I told her I didn't feel well and described my symptoms, she told me if it was as bad as I said, I should go to the hospital. I was shocked to hear her say that, and then pure, solid, panic set in; I was terrified to miss basketball practice. My coach was not one to accept questionable excuses for missing a practice. There was no way in the world I wanted to cross her. In tears, I told my mom I had to go to practice.

She was not happy that I was making that choice, and she forbade me to drive if my chest hurt. I begged her; I pleaded; she stood firm. No. I asked if she could take me, but she said no because her work and my school were in opposite directions.

I did what a lot of kids do. When one parent says no, you call the other. I called my dad and told him what was happening. He agreed to come pick me up and take me to and from practice. He and I agreed: "No pain; no gain." But he also warned me that if my symptoms got worse, I needed to call him right away. My mom made me promise to tell my coach that I was having chest pains. Yeah, like she would take it easy on me? Not hardly.

And so I went to practice and did everything I could to ignore my pain and push it out of my head. Each breath was excruciating; each catch of the basketball radiated with a dull throb that traveled down my arms to the middle of my back. When practice was over and I went to school the next day, my pain was back to "normal."

That was my first experience with that chest discomfort and pain, but it would not be my last. As a matter of fact, it would get worse as I got older. I never forgot what it felt like that first time, and eventually, when it was happening with more frequency, I included it on my earliest T-charts.

As with so many other symptoms, it seemed to ease after the Chiari malformation surgery only to return full force in 2006. This pain, in hindsight, had a direct correlation to ankylosing spondylitis and scleroderma. In 1989, I don't think either of those diseases would have been on an attending physician's radar if I had gone to the emergency room. And I'm one-hundred percent sure that my first GP would have chalked it up to hypochondria.

On the one hand, you may think I was foolish for going to basketball practice in light of the severe pain I felt, and that my parents were less than responsible, but, on the other hand, it is this same perseverance that gave me the determination to find the answers to my lifetime of pain and illness. And once I knew that I had this whole constellation of autoimmune diseases and I learned that my only hope was a stem cell transplant, you better believe I was ready to move heaven and earth to make it happen.

Sometimes it is difficult to balance patience with perseverance. How long should you wait patiently for someone to come up with a diagnosis? When is it time to kick yourself in the butt and act on your own behalf, to persevere in your search for answers. For me, I learned to balance them reasonably well; learning patience meant I could persevere; when an answer was not immediately forthcoming, I tried hard to believe that it would be just around the next corner, that I could be patient, but at the same time, I couldn't expect someone else to do it for me. I had to act. My perseverance led me to my peripheral stem cell transplant. You will identify and set as your goal whatever equals success for you.

Before I get further into this chapter I want to tell you that your point of success (that goal you are pursuing) will most likely change over time. This is often out of your control for reasons such as medical breakthroughs, new discoveries in causes and treatments, new doctors, new information acquired through your own learning, and even changes in your team. For a very long time, close to four and a half years, I knew a stem cell transplant was my best option for returning to living and working full time. But until I met Liz, it was not my identified point of success. My success point was very much goal oriented, but, at that time, it involved dying with dignity and the legacy I would leave behind. Liz is the reason my success point changed to living instead of dying; because of her I had hope and getting the stem cell transplant meant I might live. She gave me the hope and faith I needed to believe that it was possible. Pre-Liz, I knew I could never afford to pay for a transplant, and I knew the FDA wouldn't change their views on stem cell transplants for autoimmune patients like me. They wouldn't come through for me before I was too weak or too dead for the transplant to be successful. (One has to wonder why an eighty-five percent mortality rate doesn't suggest that doing the transplant sooner might be more effective. But then again I don't work for the FDA.) Liz's hope was contagious enough that it generated a new offensive line for me (my inner circle) who created the amazing fund-raising machine.

Patience

It occurs to me now how often I have used the word "patient," not just here, but throughout the book, most frequently in terms of the noun, that is, a person who is sick and under the care of a physician or waiting to get medical care, the client for medical services. However, in this chapter, I focus also on the adjective. In this usage, the word describes someone who has the ability to remain calm and in control when waiting for a long time or dealing with difficult circumstances or annoying people. A patient person is not impetuous and remains steadfast in the face of opposition or adversity. The origin of the word, according to the Merriam-Webster online dictionary, is traced back to the Latin, meaning "to suffer," and is related to a Greek word meaning "suffering." In general, the connection between the two forms appears to be that someone endures suffering without complaint.

So when I talk about being a patient patient, that is, one who exercises control while waiting for medical treatment or diagnosis, I don't mean to imply that you put up with unreasonable delays or indifferent medical staff. Knowing when you need to begin pushing back against the obstacles that stand in the way of your diagnosis or treatment is important. Knowing when you need to take an active, as opposed to a passive, role in your treatment is critical. Your medical treatment should not be something that is done to you; it should be done with you.

I'm going to take a slightly different approach to this chapter. I don't feel the need to explain the importance of patience in your health care journey. Chances are high, and I'm fairly certain, that if you are reading this book as a patient, you already know the importance of patience and have probably been to the end of your patience and back again. You certainly don't need one more voice telling you, "Be patient."

I really dislike that phrase anyway. For me, and I would imagine for you too, when it comes to medical matters and people telling me to "be patient" (even when their intentions are good), sometimes all I want to do is scream and say, "Patience be damned! I have a right to be impatient!" The admonition sometimes becomes the equivalent of telling me "Don't panic," when there is a super huge "B52" (that would be one of Hawaii's infamous flying cockroaches) in my office. If I know it is there, I'm gonna panic. Those bugs are just gross and, no matter what anyone tries to tell me, I KNOW they're big enough to eat me.

It's not that I'm always impatient when it comes to my health, but there are those times when I want the results yesterday. I even got to a point with my rheumatologist (my quarterback) that I was so tired of all the medications and the methotrexate injections that I stopped taking everything for three months. The autoimmune diseases were still progressing in spite of the medications and the injections, which were just band aids covering the symptoms.

I was both spiritually and financially broke, and I wanted a summer where I wasn't imprisoned by the cost of my medications, all of which had a side effect of some sort. My quarterback understood what I wanted, so we stopped the medications gradually. Part of me was so tired of waiting for a cure that I figured if there wasn't going to be one, then I wanted some freedom and time to just live until I couldn't anymore. I simply couldn't be a patient patient any longer. For three months I had some version of "freedom." Unfortunately, the symptoms returned bigger, better, and stronger once all the medications were completely out of my system. Damn.

So this chapter will not be me telling you how to be patient or how to persevere. Certainly, my patience failed me many times. What I would like to do is show you how I managed to maintain patience, albeit unevenly, on my journey and how I still manage it since my journey isn't over by a long shot. My hope is that you will be open to my thoughts and determine whether any or all can be of value in your medical journey. But, if not, I hope you find something to laugh about or find some comfort in the stories I will share.

Wanting A Bald Head

You and I both know a lot of people get upset over losing their hair from chemotherapy. However, I was excited—not at the prospect of chemotherapy, but of finally having a bald head. For several years I had thought about what it would be like to have a bald head. I've never been vain about my hair, and sometimes I just thought it was downright annoying. You would be surprised to know how long I had been waiting for an opportunity to shave my head. When the chance came along, I wanted the barber as soon as possible.

In 2005, after I was diagnosed with cancer, I was sitting in the doctor's office waiting for him to come in and give me the results of the biopsies, and my first thought to myself was, "Well if I need chemo, I finally get to lose my hair." Strange that I thought of that instead of the possibility of dying from cancer. At that particular time, dying wasn't exactly in my plans—yet. I just assumed I could, and would, survive the cancer.

The doctor came in, and he had the oncology psychologist with him. He sat down and introduced said counselor to me. I noticed my doctor was having a tough time making eye contact. I am one-hundred percent sure that this doctor, whom I've gotten to know quite well over the years, never likes delivering bad news to his patients (which is a good thing—I don't think any of us want doctors who enjoy that). He is one of those doctors who truly does care about his patients. So the conversation kinda went like this:

Dr. Ovary (I know, strange choice of a name, but I had to change some names and it was a "female" cancer): I have the results of your biopsies and you have stage three adenocarcinoma.

Me: Really?! Like, how many stages are there? ('Cause at this point I only remember ever hearing of four, so three must be pretty serious.)

Dr. Ovary: There are four stages and yours can progress quickly if we don't do a hysterectomy right away. You are quite young and I've asked Dr. Psych to be here to talk with you to help you understand what this all means.

Dr. Psych: I work with cancer patients all the time and will help with you get through this.

Me: Okay...

Dr. Ovary: This does mean that you won't be able to carry and deliver your own children.

Dr. Psych: This sense of loss can be overwhelming.

Me: Yeah, okay, I get that. The best part is I can go swimming whenever I want and I will save some money each month on those bulky feminine hygiene products. Any chance I will lose my hair 'cause that would be so cool?

Dr. Psych: I think I don't need to be here.

Laughter.....

Fast forward to February 2011, Sitting in Dr. Uramoto's office in Hawaii:

(Dr. Zafer Gülbaş, from Anadolu Medical Center, in Turkey, Dr. Uramoto, from Honolulu, Liz, and me)

Dr. G to Dr. U: Do you think Cristy is a good patient for the transplant?

Dr. U: Absolutely. If for no other reason because her mind is in the right place to get through it.

Dr. G to me: Are you prepared for the transplant?

Me: Oh yes! And I'm going to lose my hair. (Big smiles from me, weird looks from Dr. G, Dr. U, and Liz)

Dr. G: Is that a good thing?

I know he and the others were puzzled, but the thought of being bald has always been an exciting thing for me. No more trying to keep the frizz down, no more having to wash and blow dry my hair every morning, no more bed head, no more trying to look like everyone expects a woman to look. FREEDOM! Total and complete freedom. So knowing I was going to be able to shave my head without people constantly questioning me or making comments about how my hair looks, I moved into the classic impatient patient.

And, to be honest, it's possible in both situations I was making light of a very serious situation because it was something I wasn't quite sure of and I was maybe a little scared.

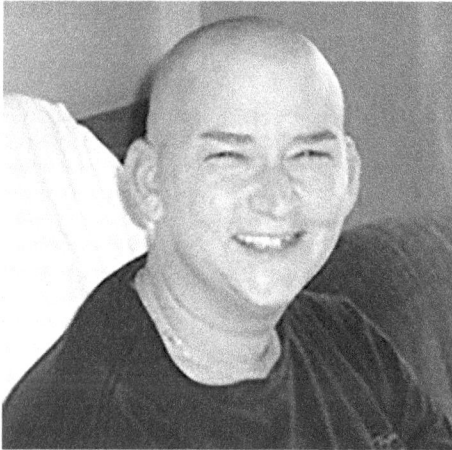

Freedom from bedhead!!

After my first two nights in the hospital in Turkey, I asked Dilek, my international patient representative (or patient advocate) at Anadolu, to get the barber to come over and shave my head. First, I really didn't feel like dealing with bed head in the hospital. Second, as anyone knows who has had chemo, the hair/head starts to hurt. You wake up in the morning with chunks of hair all over the pillow and in your mouth. It is just easier to get rid of it before it starts to fall out. One of my favorite memories of the transplant was the amazing feeling of taking my first shower bald. Liberating and free...

Disclaimer: I am in no way making light of cancer, or other reasons for chemotherapy, and the effects of such an awful enemy. I am, however, a proponent of a positive, kick-ass kinda attitude if one can get there.

While this story might be a funny example of patience and perseverance on the medical journey, I mean, really, c'mon, being impatient over getting to shave my head, that doesn't really seem to fit into such a serious topic of navigating a serious disease or diagnosis. But does it really hurt to find something trivial to laugh about? Because now I will tell you about the ugly side of impatience and how it can really "eat" away at you when your energy needs to be put toward survival.

And I have to point out that Dilek, who happily called the barber when I requested it, was a wonderful patient representative. She was always available to answer our questions and to see to our needs. She is the kind of professional patient advocate anyone would want to work with in times of crisis.

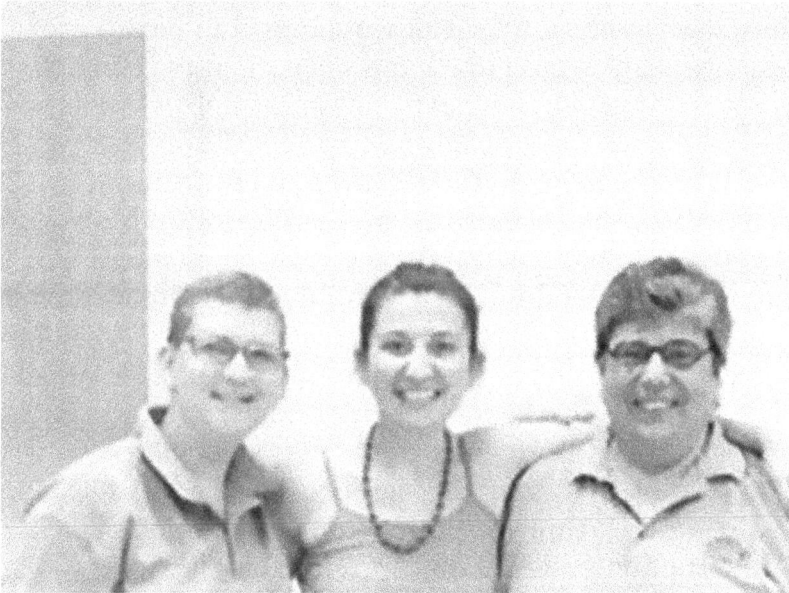

Cristy and Liz with Dilek Inci, one of the best professional patient advocates you could ever work with.

I am so glad to have found her and to have her to help me and Liz make the best decisions for my health care. She is part of what makes Anadolu work so beautifully for its patients.

Patience and Perseverance

The *One of Our Own Fund* team began fund raising on my behalf in early 2010. The money wasn't something that consumed my thoughts until I had two viable options for my transplant: Bangkok or Turkey. Then the money mattered because my newly identified point of success was getting the transplant—it was my only hope. The *One of Our Own Fund* team tirelessly raised money from strangers and donated their own money to get me where I needed to go so I could live. Much of the early money they raised went to pay my outstanding medical bills, and when I found out how much the transplant would really cost, I realized that it would be impossible for them to raise all of the money I would need. I didn't believe we could do it without one seriously rich donor or asking someone I knew for a loan. In order to secure a loan, it would need to be a personal loan. No bank would touch me since I hadn't had enough recovery time between paying off prior medical debts and needing funds for the transplant.

With the help of WorldMed Assist, a medical tourism company, we had decided the best option for the transplant was the Anadolu Medical Center, near Istanbul, Turkey, a non-profit hospital affiliated with Johns Hopkins Medicine. It was a rare, but fortunate coincidence that Dr. Gülbaş traveled to Honolulu for a conference and agreed to consult with me and my rheumatologist to determine whether I was a good candidate for a stem cell transplant. Of course, you've already read that he agreed I was, and we began to try to put everything in motion for it to really happen. This meant not only raising funds for the transplant itself, but also paying for our transportation to Turkey and our living expenses for a minimum of two months for the procedure and for follow-up care until I was able to come home. I really was going to need a loan; otherwise we would have to give up hope.

I watched the days disappear as the time drew closer to when Liz and I needed to leave for Turkey. We needed to be prepared with a down payment of half of the estimated costs when we arrived at the hospital with the remainder due upon discharge. Unfortunately, the *One of Our Own Fund* had only raised about fifty percent of the costs. Where would the other half come from in such a short time?

I am somewhat embarrassed with what I am about to tell you. But this is what happens when impatience really sets in and your mind is consumed by desperate thoughts and a creeping hopelessness. My family had known for at least a year I was trying to raise money for my transplant. In fact, they had come to the fundraiser that was held in Maryland. Some members of my family really surprised me with how generous they were and still are. Yet, the one person whom I believed could really help me out with a loan, my mother, hadn't said a word or even offered to help. For months I updated her on the number of donations and the total amount raised. She would ask, or I would openly share, my concern over how much more was needed and how I would get it. We even talked about those people who might consider loaning me the money.

My heart grew increasingly heavy because she never mentioned loaning me the money, and I was scared to death to come right out and ask her. It is a hard thing to have to go back to mom when you are forty years old. So time continued to tick off on the clock. In the back of my mind, I continued to wonder why my mom hadn't offered to help, and I would find myself worrying and getting very anxious. I told Liz repeatedly that I wasn't going to go through with the transplant. That if we couldn't pay for it, I couldn't do it. We couldn't just show up in Turkey and pay them the fifty percent down payment if we couldn't pay the rest after the treatment. I was losing hope, but we didn't cancel the trip or the appointment—we just kept praying for a miracle.

Intellectually, I knew, with two weeks left before the transplant start date, anything was possible. My spirit and heart grew increasingly impatient. It was time to reach a decision: I was either going to Turkey or I was staying home to die. Finally, just days before Liz and I were to leave for Anadolu, I called my mom. In tears and having trouble catching my breath, I asked her to please, please consider giving me a loan. And through her tears, she told me that she and my stepdad had talked about it and I should know it was never something they would not do for me. They had always planned on loaning me the difference in the money.

Lesson: When you're at the end of your rope with patience and it seems like persevering is out of the question, ask the question you most need the answer to.

Lesson: People can't read your mind; try to be as clear as you can when you are looking for help. I spent probably two months beating around the bush when I talked to my mom about the money and a loan. And my mom never thought that I didn't "just" know she would be there to help.

You may be asking yourself how this demonstrates the need for patience. In my increasing level of impatience over the money, I found myself begging Liz, and some others on the *One of Our Own Fund* team, to ask for money from others when the timing wasn't right or the relationship wasn't there. Had I been patient with my mom and just asked her for help, I wouldn't be the reason Liz faced strained relationships with some of her long-time acquaintances.

The two stories I chose to share with you are ones that might provide a picture of other aspects of your medical journey aside from the typical stories associated with waiting for test results, waiting for doctors' appointments, waiting to have a test done, or simply just waiting for a diagnosis. Sometimes we need to step back and take a look at how the waiting for diagnosis, test results, appointments, and so on, can lead us to become impatient in other areas. I would give anything to travel back in time and be able to slap my hand over my mouth all of those times I was short, or rude with various health care professionals. As we know hindsight is always 20/20. If only I could have predicted the success of my transplant then, of course, being patient would have been a whole lot easier.

Summary

In the next chapter on sustainability I will share with you how I was able to persevere and patiently stay the course for at least sixty percent of the time. If there is one thing I want to convey to you about being patient, it is to let yourself have moments where you either verbalize or visualize your impatience. In other words, give yourself the time and place to talk out loud (to someone or not) or write all the things causing you to become impatient. Give yourself time to feel; and no matter what you are feeling there is no right or wrong. If you feel angry because the results are taking too long, be angry. How you express the anger is key.

One of my favorite ways to express my frustration with having to be patient, or waiting, was to get in my car and drive, screaming for as loud and as long as I could. (I recommend that you keep the windows up and always travel at the posted speed. When I screamed once at a red light I got some very funny looks.)

And although I really dislike the phrase, "Be patient," I will tell you that when faced with a health care crisis, remaining as patient as you can with your team will help you persevere and survive the journey.

Just Remember

- Balance patience with perseverance: be prepared to wait, but know when you need to push for action.

- Identify your success point and go for it.

- Recognize that your success point can change.

- Find something to laugh about.

- Investigate every conceivable avenue for achieving your success point.

- Ask the question(s) you most need the answer(s) to.

- Try to be as clear as you can when you are looking for help.

- Find a harmless outlet for your frustrations and anger. Don't take it out on your team (your doctors, your support network, or your care giver).

S.T.E.P.S. in Action:
Perseverance and Patience

When being the patient patient doesn't work, you have to persevere (even if it isn't what the doctor had in mind). Let me paint you a picture of what it was like in Turkey for the transplant.

At first, it wasn't too hard to remain patient while in the transplant unit. Ativan was my friend, and I believe it was an essential element for success of transplant. And even with my "friend" on board, I still had bad days, especially after March 21, 2011 (my re-birth day) when Dr. Gülbaş brought the results of my blood tests.

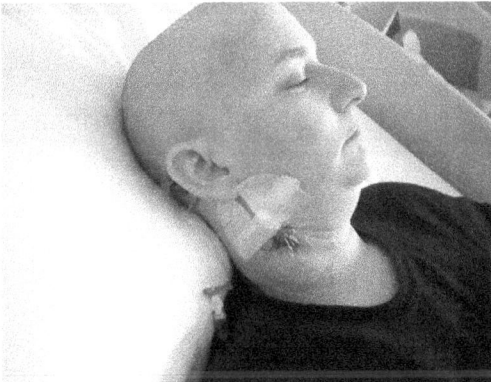

The jugular port, through wihich the stem cells were transfused.

Once I heard the awesome news that my liver and kidney functions were normal, all I wanted was to get that damn port out of my jugular vein. (The worst part of that port was the machine alarm that would go off if I moved a certain way. There was an all-day parade of nurses coming in to turn it off.) I also wanted the freedom to pee without collecting it in a bottle to make certain my output precisely matched my input each and every day. (Yes, Liz kept a daily log of each drop of liquid that entered my body.). I wanted so badly to sleep late once in a while instead of having that six o'clock wakeup when the first of my nurses arrived to hang super-sized bags of prednisone and poke me with hypodermic needles, especially the ones with Neupogen which left huge black and blue bruises on my arms.

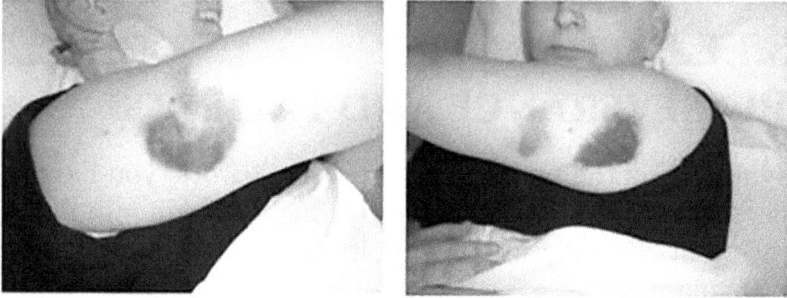

The bruises from neupogen injections.

As long as I was in the transplant ward, Dr. Gülbaş controlled my eventual release date. Even if I had the strength to do it, there was no sneaking in or out of the ward because security cameras were everywhere, and every door was securely monitored and locked. I would have needed the secret code to be let in or let out. Yes, there were times I compared it to a prison or detention center. Eventually, I truly appreciated why the transplant center was managed this way, but honestly, right there and right then, all I wanted was to go home.

Finally the day came. My first reprieve: April 5, 2011, about two weeks after the transplant, when Dr. Gülbaş gave the okay for me to exit the secure facility and return to our hotel room. (Was it really only two weeks? It seemed like an eternity.) My freedom, though, was limited because of the serious danger of infection. I wasn't going to get to run out and start painting Istanbul red every night. I still needed a pretty sterile environment, and I needed to follow-up with Dr. Gülbaş once a week. But it was a blessed start. The hospital escort came to get me in a wheel chair to take Liz and me back to our hotel, which was right there on the campus of the medical center.

We had to go outside and follow a walking path from the medical center to the hotel. It felt so liberating when the hospital doors swung open and our escort pushed me outside. It was winter in Turkey and we were getting a light snowfall. The air felt crisp and cold, even through my layers of protective clothing. I wanted to breathe in that fresh, cold air and to catch a snowflake on my tongue, but my surgical mask had other ideas, filtering and warming the air I breathed and stopping my tongue dead in its tracks. In spite of that, it truly felt like I was experiencing a newness and a whole new brightness of life. I was free. I was getting healthy.

So, yeah, there you have it. Kind of one of those perfect movie scenes: cue the music and fade. Right? Right. It lasted about a week.

I still wanted to go home. To my house. I wanted to be able to pick up my phone and hear my dad's voice without crying because I missed him so much. I wanted to start planning for when my mom could come visit. I wanted to start planning visits from my friend, Jenne (who promised me if I survived the transplant she would come see me), and my cousin, Abby (who lost her sister and father to cancer two years apart). I wanted to be outside and see the ocean—my ocean in Honolulu. But no, we had to patiently persevere and stay the course for the first 100 days post-transplant. We were left with eighty-some days before we could go home.

One week later, I had my first follow-up visit with Dr. Gülbaş. All the labs were great, my blood cell counts were doing exactly what they needed to do, and so I did what I do naturally. I used my sense of humor to try and convince him to let me fly home. He did a great job of seeing my humor and raising the stakes, also through humor, telling Liz and me we could go home as soon as we found a nonstop flight from Istanbul to Honolulu. However, one should never underestimate my resolve.

With a smile and a new determination I set out to learn everything I could on flying routes, airlines, people with private jets, costs of private jets. (There's that education thing again.) But alas, I had to surrender to the fact that a very disgustingly rich person with a private jet fleet was not going to donate their services or "necessities" just because I wanted to be in my own house, my own island "mansion."

By the second follow-up visit with Dr. Gülbaş, one week later, not only was I very homesick but Liz was hitting the breaking point, too. (To this day we do not travel away from home for more than two weeks at a time.) So I put Plan B into action; when humor doesn't work, bring on the tears. And it worked like a charm. Not only was I crying to go home, but Liz was following suit, almost as if we had planned the whole thing. I wish I could say the tears were all acting, but not even one of them was fake. We needed to go home. Intellectually, I understood I had gone through a traumatic medical procedure and my body was in need of a long period of recovery, but, emotionally, I was getting depressed.

Dr. Gülbaş sternly reminded us of the importance of my first one-hundred days, and I promised—cross my heart and hope to die—well, no, just cross my heart—to fly home with only my eyes visible. Meaning, I would remain covered head to toe with a skull cap to keep my awesome bald head germ free, a face mask to protect me from inhaled germs, long sleeves and pants, and gloves to make sure I didn't touch those public, disgusting germ-laden surfaces and then touch my face. Dr. Gülbaş explained risks involved with flying and Liz promised she would find a way for me to fly business class or first class all the way home. Finally, we reached a compromise if Liz and I could find a flight with only one stop, he would agree to let us go home in five days if my chest x-ray was clear and all of my labs were holding steady.

Finally, my second reprieve was a reality. The impatient patient found an itinerary that Dr. Gülbaş approved even though there were three stops involved. We flew from Istanbul to Frankfurt, then to San Francisco, and finally Honolulu. He approved it because Liz, the persevering priest, worked long and hard with the amazing folks at United Airlines to get us relatively short layovers, airport assistance, Premier Club access between flights (so my exposure to the general population in the airports was limited), and upgrades using our miles all the way home.

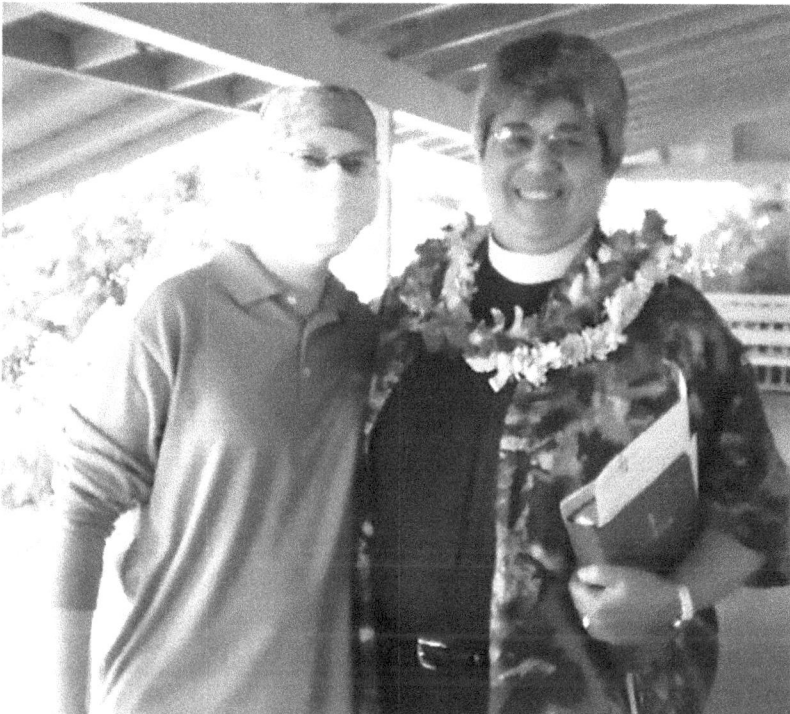

Celebrating her "first" Easter with Liz

Once home, we were extremely careful to stick to everything we had promised Dr. Gülbaş. There was no way we were going to undo all of the good he had done for me.

The moral of this story here, folks, is not if you cry, you'll get your way. But crying does help.

Chapter 6—Step 5: Sustainability

Sometimes the questions are complicated and the answers simple.
Dr. Seuss

As I was putting my thoughts to paper regarding the *5 S.T.E.P.S.*, I struggled at times with the notion of where topics associated with patience and perseverance stop and sustainability takes over. Blurred lines, or shades of grey, if you will. In order to clarify the difference between these two steps, I think of the concept of sustainability as a means of managing both patience and perseverance, of achieving the balance that is so necessary for me as a patient enduring the journey through an oftentimes difficult and indifferent medical maze.

Sustainability, the fifth step in *5 S.T.E.P.S.* is all about you and what you need to take care of and protect your body, mind, and spirit. Sustainability for patients like you (and me) involves deep thought and reflection to determine what you need in your life that will help you keep going day after day after day. I don't mean determining what you need in terms of medications or therapy or anything related to treatment and diagnosis. I mean what you need psychologically to establish and maintain a frame of mind that says, "I will not give up. I don't care what you throw at me, I will not quit."

In the previous four steps, I talked about being your own patient advocate and what that looks like in your relationships with your doctors, your significant others, your family, your friends, and colleagues. I talk about the importance of education not just for you, but also for those on your team who need to be "in the know" as well. In this chapter I will share with you the things I had to do for me in order to ensure I had enough "fuel" in the tank to keep living.

Sustainability is defined as a method of harvesting or using a resource so that the resource is not depleted or permanently damaged. I rather like one of the definitions of the word sustainable, which is, "to be used without being used up;" there are times in your medical journey when you will begin to feel "used up," wondering where in the world you will find the strength or the will to keep going. When I see or hear the word I automatically think about gardening or farming. I had a friend who used to say, "If you're green, you're growing. If you're ripe, you rot." And to some extent that is true. As living creatures, we need to sustain ourselves and find ways to grow even when it seems the weight of our health care battles is more than we can bear. In each of the other chapters I have talked about ways to become engaged in your own health care. My goal is to keep you active in your own care so you don't become stagnant. Being stagnant in health care can essentially mean, as my friend would say, you rot. Being a patient patient does not mean being a passive patient. There is no better way to sustain yourself then to find a balance between waiting calmly and recognizing when to act on something urgent in your life and circumstances.

I spent almost a year in rapid decline prior to my transplant. This made it very difficult to do the things I had previously enjoyed as hobbies or pastimes, like walking and swimming and snorkeling. For a while, I spent my sick leave feeling guilty for not working and beating myself up for being lazy. Since childhood, I had been conditioned to believe that because I required more sleep and naps than others my age, I was a lazy child. I frequently felt useless, which would then lead me down the path of hopelessness, struggling, and sometimes failing, to maintain the will power and drive to get to the transplant. As you read in the previous chapter, there were times I saw it as an impossible goal and wondered why I was even imagining it for myself.

As much as I wanted to believe others could sustain me or make me feel valued, it was impossible for others to do what I could not do for myself. The simple answer to this complicated issue was that I was responsible for sustaining myself: body, mind, and spirit.

Sustainability Through Therapy

The single, most important thing I have done to sustain myself was to begin working with a therapist. I was first introduced to the idea of a counselor when I was in high school and for most of my life before relocating to Hawaii, I spent a lot of time trying to find the "right" therapist for me. I do not want to minimize the idea of therapy, and finding the right fit is important. I know a lot of people who avoid going into therapy simply because of the stigma— you know, "If you're seeing a therapist, you must be crazy." For a very long time, I spent a great deal of energy trying to "spin" or justify going for professional therapy. And, oddly enough, I spent even longer hiding from my counselors the fact that I felt depressed and had some significant anxiety issues; after all, you would think that was why I was seeing them, wouldn't you?

Imagine this scenario: I go to the therapist. She asks if I'm depressed. I respond with a twenty-minute diatribe explaining why I was justified in feeling what I was feeling. Counselor after counselor after.... You get the picture. I refused to be on drugs for depression or anxiety. I did not want to deal with the stigma. And if I was going to be on anti-depressants, I didn't want anyone to know. Even after giving in to taking them, I had my prescription filled in a different town from where I lived and worked because I was afraid people would think I was incompetent. How could a teacher and coach be clinically depressed? What would happen to my job if my boss found out, and how would my parents and family treat me? Would they be ashamed?

I am here to tell you there is no shame in taking medication for imbalances that are cognitive in nature. I have a reasonably long history of clinical depression and now, since the transplant, chemotherapy-induced ADHD. I take drugs for both. And as I've matured, I have evolved, coming to recognize these drugs as my friends.

Let's get real here. I have suffered with illness all my life. I grew up enduring sometimes excruciating pain all over my body. Living like this is bound to build up and begin to weigh a person down. Taking care of my mind is just as important as fighting for the right treatment for my body. My one piece of advice on developing a healthy mind in the face of your medical crises is don't do it half-assed. Give your mind the same effort as you give your body. You are worth it. It wasn't until I moved to Hawaii that I finally got it right in regards to my mental health. Instead of window-shopping for the right counselor, I needed to go inside and try them on. It's like my mom used to say when we were shoe shopping: if the shoes hurt your feet when you first put them on, don't buy them. When meeting with a therapist for the first time, you know in the first ten minutes if the shoes fit. There is no harm in finishing the session and not going back. And I strongly encourage you to only keep paying for a service if it feels comfortable to you.

Before I actually made my first appointment with my psychiatrist in Hawaii I tried to learn (there's that education thingy again) as much as I could about several doctors before choosing one. I surfed the 'net looking for reviews and I asked family and friends for recommendations. I was pretty certain I was making a good selection before I even met the psychiatrist in person. I ended up staying with this doctor for five years and only recently switched to a duo arrangement to care for my mental health (a psychiatrist and a therapist).

Talking to another human every week or so where I don't have to worry about being judged for my word choice or tone gives me the strength I need to be a better person for all of my interpersonal relationships. Through counseling I also was able to focus on new hobbies and interests that could sustain me on my health care journey without zapping all of my energy or consuming my "awake" time, that is, my time not spent in bed. During one session, it occurred to me that I would love to try planting a small garden at home. Even now, I'm like, "Where did that come from?" But twenty minutes twice a day outside landscaping and gardening provided me with so much joy. I loved watching my little tree with only two tiny twigs branching off its trunk grow from twenty-four inches tall to over ten feet in two years. The first time Liz and I were able to pick tomatoes and Japanese cucumbers was amazing. The garden and the gardening made me happy. I didn't need validation from another human because I was receiving validation from watching living things grow and knowing that my hands had started it all. It brought me joy.

Sustainability Through Faith

I would be remiss if I didn't share with you some aspects of my faith in the conversation about sustainability. And trust me, some days my faith was the only thing I had that gave me the patience to stay the course. Each of you will need to examine the role of faith in your life and the extent to which it is important and the extent to which you take comfort from it. I don't want to dictate how you should think or feel or participate in faith-based groups; I simply want to share my story of my faith and how it helped me.

When you walk into my office at UH the first thing you will see after noticing the very green-ness of my walls (it's called "Nifty Green;" clever, eh?) is a banner that stretches the length of my far wall that says: "Faith is daring the soul to go beyond what the eyes can see." The words come from William Newton Clark, a nineteenth century theologian and professor at Colgate Theological Seminary, and they resonate with me. My faith is strong. My faith is deep. I wholeheartedly believe in the power of the Holy Spirit. I believe She is the most powerful force I am connected to and because of Her, I am able to persevere and sustain my life.

If you examine the previous two sentences, you may think you can determine the depths of my religion or spirituality. And that's okay to do; I encourage it. Because when you examine them, for a brief period of time you, then, are thinking about a force (or whatever word you want to substitute) greater than yourself.

Medical journeys are hard and long. And no matter how simple or how complicated the journey may seem to you, it is very tiring. A fundamental reason I was able to sustain myself during my journey is because, for a time, I did not allow my health to be the most significant focal point in my life on a daily basis, at least until it consumed more than twelve hours a day. Oh, it was there, every single day, all day long. I just chose not to allow it to be front and center if I could help it. Of course, the more my health deteriorated the more difficult it was to focus on other things.

And that is the moral of this story. Well, kinda. You see, through the years I've been to a lot of churches. Some I joined, some I didn't. Some I liked; some I didn't. But something—for me, the Holy Spirit—kept driving me back to the concepts of faith and religion. As a trained social studies teacher, I have found myself, both personally and professionally, in places where I've studied and/or reflected on various aspects of world religions. And with all I have learned and all I have taught about the diverse religions of this world, I can say, without any doubt, a power greater than I has sustained me throughout my medical journey. I believe there is a reason I'm still walking this earth and I continue to ponder what those reasons are.

For whatever reason, I have found the power of my own daily prayer and meditation to be life giving. And for me, not just because my partner is a priest, I find that going to a chapel regularly, and, more importantly, taking time each day to meditate or pray, I can find inner peace so that I am sustaining my spirit. My physical health would not be where it is today if I did not nurture my spirit. My spirit is just as important to my overall success as my mind and body are. Your spirit needs to be important, too. I'm sure it doesn't need to look exactly like mine, but find something that brings calm into your life and gives you hope. Dare your soul to go beyond what your eyes can see.

Sustainability and Social Media

Being face-to-face with people while you're sick isn't always easy. Lord knows there were days I did NOT want anyone to see what I looked like. Aside from that, the physical energy it took to get showered, dressed, and drive somewhere would require me to have to pull off the road at some point and take a power nap. I'm serious. Enter the power of social media. Facebook is a saving grace for me, just as Twitter would become later on after the transplant (details to come in my next book). Between Facebook, texting, and email, I could interact with people sometimes almost immediately. Other times I could read emails and respond when I had the energy. I didn't have to worry about people on the other end of the telephone hearing pain or fatigue in my voice. I could just communicate as me. Nothing more, nothing less.

I also used social media to stay connected with my students and educational and professional interests. I developed new relationships with folks without ever letting on I was sick. And when you make a connection with someone because of mutual interests, you get a sense that they are learning about you because they want to, not because they feel sorry for you because you are sick.

In the two months I was in Turkey for the transplant, social media and email were my major avenues for staying connected with the outside world. It was through these means that I was able to stay in touch with my dad. That daily connection through a computer sustained me on days when I was really homesick or worried that my body might reject my own stem cells. I could sense my dad's strength through each and every email. I can't even imagine what it was like for transplant patients before computers, Internet, and cell phones. I definitely would have required more Ativan.

But I have to tell you, my real social media adventure began with Twitter!

While in Turkey for my transplant, Liz and I fell in love with MasterChef Turkey. Now keep in mind it was all in Turkish with no subtitles, but the inflection in the voices and non-verbal body language of the judges provided a wonderful escape from the intense chemotherapy and isolation. Of course, there were only two television channels in English, CNN International and BBC world news, so we just had to surf the Turkish language channels for a break from the news.

Fast forward to April 2011: I was back home but still very weak and needed to be in isolation with the exception of twenty minutes of walking a day. The need to guard against infection was critical. But then, Liz and I began to see promos for MasterChef, Season Two.

It began airing on Monday and Tuesday nights right before Hell's Kitchen. My interest in MasterChef only grew stronger as my need to change my cooking and eating habits increased after the transplant. So when the show got down to the final eight contestants, I decided to see if I could connect with Ben Starr, who was one of the contestants I most admired. I set up a Twitter account and sent my first tweet to Ben, "We love you in da islands." Less than twenty-four hours later, Ben tweeted back, "I love y'all in da islands, too." I ended up tweeting back and forth with four of the semi-finalists, Jennifer Behm, who later was the season two winner, Adrien Nieto, who placed second, and Tracy Kontos and Ben Starr, both of whom were among the semi-finalists.

Eventually, those four chefs, along with Christian Collins and Chef Graham Elliot, would become members of my social network *'ohana*. The original Twitter Four, as I call them, agreed to come to Hawaii to cook for Family Promise and Yo!House in January, 2012. Family Promise supports homeless families with children, and Yo!House is an organization that helps homeless teens on the island of Oahu. They prepared the meals at Liz's parish kitchen at St. Clement, feeding more than one hundred people while they were there.

For me, raising the money to get these television celebrity chefs to come to Hawaii was a way for me to pay it forward. I had been so fortunate, but there were so many others who needed help. It wasn't until the chefs arrived on-island that they learned about my illnesses and the stem cell transplant. I had not shared any of that history with them.

In 2013, Ben, Adrien, and Christian returned to Hawaii to make our new condo livable. Because my immune system was still new and vulnerable, it was not safe for me to live in a home with carpeting and wallpaper from 1976; they came to Honolulu and gutted the condo, laid new flooring, and painted every wall.

Their friendship and support, which was initiated through social media, has helped to sustain me during my recovery. Chef Graham Elliot has continued to support me via Twitter and together we are trying to get into shape. With his encouragement, I continue to build up my stamina by taking longer, faster walks (slowed only by my four-legged friend, Leah Kessler, who is almost ten years old now). I'm thinking Graham Elliot should be President; he's that awesome.

Sustainability and Your Pets

And speaking of Leah, the final sustaining force in my life has been my interactions with living creatures. And I don't just mean humans. It also refers to the animals that share my life, my pets. Being sick can be isolating.

My relationships with creatures has always been strong, to the point that once I met a German Shepard with K-9 training who laid down by my feet and requested a belly rub, much to the surprise of his owner. But it was no surprise that once I started to experience my health decline post-hysterectomy that Sidney (my feline companion of eighteen years who passed over the Rainbow Bridge in 2008) was acutely aware of my illnesses. She was a major player on my offensive line and a direct link to my sustainability. Sidney was exactly what I needed because I was responsible for her daily care. Knowing Sidney relied on me to provide her with her basic needs (which cost money) I was even more determined to keep working and not give up on finding ways to fix my health. It might sound crazy that a cat could motivate a human to fight harder to stay employed and be healthy, but for those of you who are pet lovers, you know they are our children. With all Sidney had endured with me throughout her life, I wasn't about to stop providing for her.

While I was extremely sad when Sidney passed away, I felt guilty because I was also somewhat relieved. I was relieved that I wouldn't have to expend the energy to keep up with litter box cleaning and sweeping up litter tracks since she was gone. It also meant a financial savings that I could shift to my own needs. However, it didn't matter how many positives I could find in Sidney's death, they just didn't outweigh the impact a pet has on sustaining your own life. In less than two months I realized how joy-less my home was. I found myself missing the "smack" across my face each morning telling me to get out of bed and serve Sidney her milk. (If I ignored the "smack," everything from my dresser would invariably start falling to the floor.) I'm telling you, Sidney gave me a reason to get up every day. Without her, it would have been real easy to stay in bed, pull the covers up, and wait to die. And that, my friend, is not good.

I eventually adopted two rescued kittens, because, according to Liz, felines need to be adopted in pairs and I needed to experience life with kittens. (Sidney was almost a year old when I adopted her.) So, in December 2008, just in time to experience their first Christmas tree, Bristol and Bailey Kessler came home. The joys of new parenthood once again added a much-needed dynamic and energy to my home and once again I was forced to remove myself from the prone position on a daily basis. Being at least a little bit mobile and active plays an important role in sustaining yourself for the long health care battle. This, my friend, is good.

As 2009 was rolling along, my health was declining at a rapid rate. I was still living on my own and trying to maintain my energy levels. It was growing increasingly difficult. Part of who I am is my ability to be very self-aware. When I seem to be a little less energetic or motivated, I have a tendency not to get out of the house as often I would like to. Try not to misunderstand here, I wasn't spiraling into a depression; I have never been someone who stays inside all the time, but I do experience times when I tend to become very intrapersonal and wait for someone to invite me to do something before I go out. During this time period I was still leaving the house to go to work and to make all of my doctors' appointments. I still went grocery shopping and to church, but I wasn't feeling as moved to get outside for my walking and beach time.

So I did what any sane, unhealthy person would do, I adopted a dog. Or, rather, Leah adopted me. I saw a photo of Leah online and the brown markings around her face made her look like she had a permanent smile. I knew right then and there she was destined to be a Kessler. In August, 2009, Leah Kessler came home. Talk about sustainability, when a doggie has to go potty and you live in a condo, you go out and walk. Come hell or high water, Leah's face would be six inches from my face every morning between 6:00 and 6:30 a.m. to get my butt out of bed.

When my sick leave first began, I was so worn out and worn down that being able to sleep and not engage with people was a great relief (no offense, humans). But by month two I would read emails from work and feel so "out of it" that I felt like I was losing touch with things that had been an integral part of my life for six years.

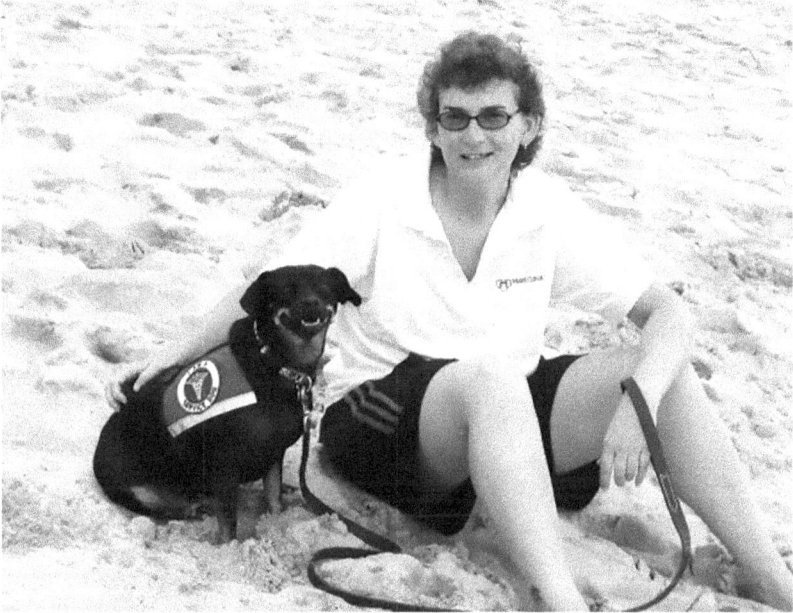

Cristy with her smiling dog, Leah

And so it began; I began talking and singing to our pets. All day, every day I would make up silly songs, talk to them like they really understood (and maybe they did). They are so important to me, and I believe I am important to them because when I am out of town they mope around until I come home. Even now as I write this, I really don't know how to express how important my pets were to sustaining me on those very low, dark days.

Sustainability and Follow-Up with Your Doctors

No matter what you have been through, no matter how close you came to death, you can never find the ways to thank the doctors who made a difference for you in your search for survival.

I cannot say enough about Dr. Uramoto and what she did that led to my stem cell transplant. She opened the door to my future--a future in which I would live and contribute to others in some way--perhaps through this book.

And Dr. Gülbaş? There are no words. How do you thank someone for saving your life? What can you ever do to repay the kindness that a doctor of his expertise offered. Yes, I know, he was paid handsomely for his services at a top-notch, international medical facility, but the gift I got is far more valuable than anything I could have gotten otherwise. As I see it, he is an angel who came into my life when I needed one the most. If my experience can contribute to the medical community's understanding of how autoimmune diseases can be served by stem cell transplant, then I am more than happy to make that

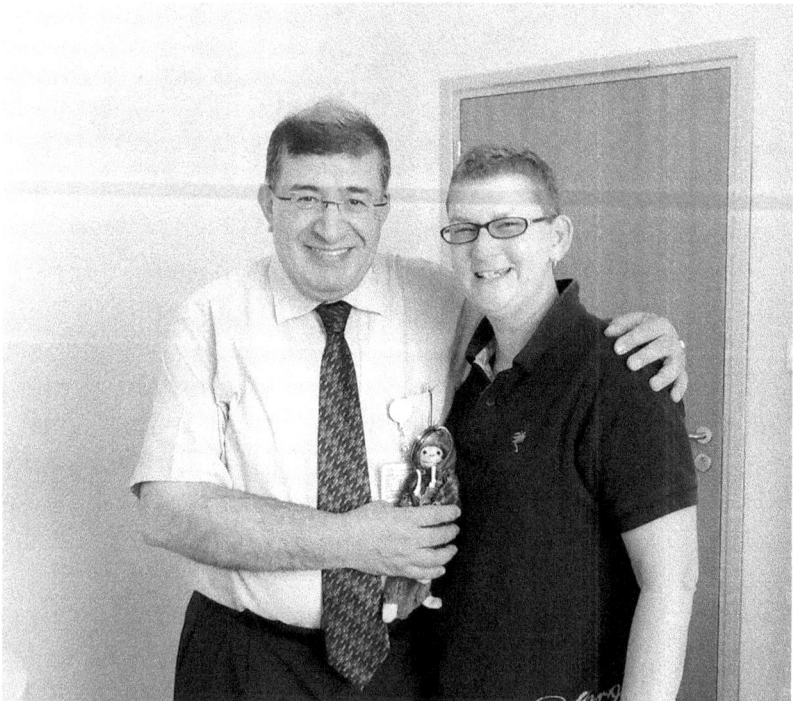

Dr Gülbaş and Cristy: 1 year follow-up visit. Even Dr. G was happy to see Woot, Cristy's noisy little traveling companion.

contribution. I can only hope that the medical community in the United States is paying attention.

Summary

In my view, sustainability throughout your medical journey is the most important step. The previous four steps matter, but unless you are active in self-sustainability, those efforts won't matter much. I think of it in terms of needing to sustain my mind and spirit during the time when my body was quitting so I didn't give up and I was ready to meet a new success point when I found it. If you take nothing else away from this book, aside from catching a glimpse of my quirky sense of humor, I hope you will find at least one thing you can make time for every day that makes you feel joy.

Pre-transplant, I enjoyed my gardening, my social media connections, my pets, and, yes, my therapy (but that was only once a week). Many of those things brought me a glimpse of hope, pre-transplant, and, if I can, I still make time for them every single day and therapy once a week. Unfortunately, I had to swap gardening for cooking for two reasons: we moved to a condo and didn't have a yard to speak of, and I had to learn to manage and meet the dietary regulations that were recommended post-transplant.

I strongly encourage you to find your avenue to calm, to hope, and to sustainability. Be the advocate for your own mind and spirit just as you would your body. It matters; you matter.

Just Remember

- Find a balance between waiting calmly and recognizing when to act on something urgent in your life and circumstances.

- You are responsible for sustaining your body, mind, and spirit.

- Give your mind the same effort as you give your body. There is no more shame in taking medications for your mind than in taking them for your body.

- Dare your soul to go beyond what your eyes can see.

- Take advantage of social media to maintain outside connections.

- Find ways to pay it forward.

- Find a reason to get out of bed every day.

- Find at least one thing you can make time for every day that makes you feel joy.

S.T.E.P.S. in Action: Sustainability

How in the heck does one really sustain herself when she has to be in another country, half a world away, for two months? (We originally were scheduled for three months, but that was before we cried to come home.) Even while I was in Turkey, all I knew and was able to do was fall back on the four things I've described in this book, plus one additional vice I will talk about shortly. Of course, I couldn't pack my therapist or pets in my suitcase to bring along, but I knew they would be there for me later.

Fortunately for me, I have the best person in my life to help raise up my faith and who is also a great listener; actually she is quite an amazing counselor in her own right, and that is Liz. Liz was more than my partner; she was my connection to my faith. Aside from what I do daily to stay connected to the Holy Spirit through private prayer and meditation, having a priest in tow meant together we could celebrate communion. We took advantage of the daily office from the Book of Common Prayer; we shared our favorite readings of scripture; and we prayed. We prayed really, really hard every day.

Being in Turkey, a traditional Islamic country, also opened the door for us to do some research and reading about Islam. There are no words to describe the beauty of the call to prayer. From where Anadolu is located, it was almost as if you could hear the call in surround sound from all the minarets throughout the city. Spectacular and awe-inspiring.

One aspect of life in Turkey that totally caught Liz and me by surprise was the way dogs are treated. It had never occurred to us that there were places in the world with feral canine communities. Liz and I were familiar with feral cat communities, because they are common in Honolulu, but such communities of dogs are either non-existent or simply not very common. We really didn't expect to see the sheer number of dogs who roamed the fields and areas around the hospital. Surprisingly, this proved to be beneficial for sustaining my relationship with creature companions.

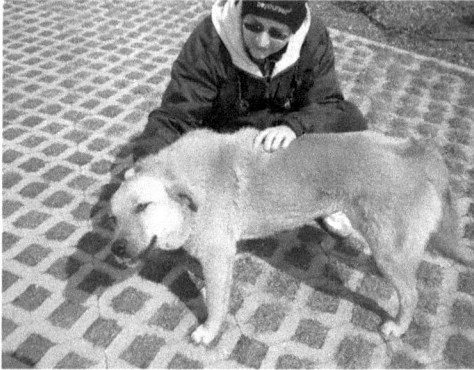

Cristy with Lexi

Within two days of arriving at Anadolu, Liz and I made friends with Lexi and King George. Lexi was a Turkish sheep dog with such an amazing, gentle demeanor. Every day Lexi waited for us to bring him leftovers from breakfast and he often napped under our hotel room window. Lexi seemed to know we always had dog treats, bones, and dog toys that Liz picked up from the local market.

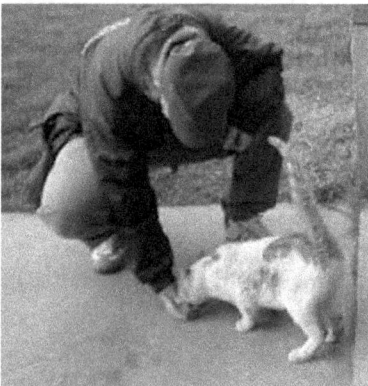

Cristy with King George, one tough, but lovable tomcat.

We befriended an orange cat that we named King George. George because when I asked Liz what to name him, that was the first name that came to her mind. King for quite a different reason. He hadn't been neutered and had one of the biggest sets of cojones we've ever seen on a cat. Clearly, he wielded some power in his feline community, because he was unscarred and unmangled, so we guessed that no other tomcat had bested him in a fight. Georgie took to trotting over to us when we walked through his territory and he heard me shake the container of kitty treats. And he always dove right in. Sometimes he followed us to the end of his territory; other times, typically catlike, he ignored us and continued to eat as we departed. With a bath and some good brushing, he would be an absolutely beautiful cat. Even with his rough, wild exterior, he was friendly and gentle and really loved rolling on his back looking for a tummy rub.

I can't understate the importance of Facebook and email while we were in Turkey. Twitter wasn't quite on my radar yet and Skype ended up being a really hard thing for me to do. Any time I Skyped with my dad (even when we didn't have the picture video working), or Jim and Sharon, or my mom, there was something about the sound of their voices and/or seeing them would leave me in the world of "what ifs" once we hung up. I got all choked up because my mind would go to THAT place—the place where I obsessed that I may never see them again. So without needing to actually talk about it, Liz and I began to limit Skype. We did, however keep Skyping with Phil and Mary Lou (our house/pet sitters) so we could see our pets and they could hear our voices. That was pretty cool, actually. Funny how I could manage the contact with our pets but struggled with managing contact with the people who meant so much to me.

Facebook played a vital role in keeping me connected to the One Of Our Own team from around the world. Through Facebook, I could always find a friend who was awake somewhere in the world who I could chat with during my sleepless nights. I was able to connect with Sandy, my longest and dearest friend. I specifically came to rely on chatting with Jenne and Sonya who could make me laugh even when I was having a very bad day. Those two really kept my spirits high. And being able to stay in touch with former students, like Lisa, gave me daily bursts of hope. I'm still amazed Jenne found a way to mail fresh Hershey's licorice to us after she saw my Facebook post about Turkish pizza coming with corn as a topping whether you order it or not. Thank you, Facebook; you sustained me through a very difficult time.

So that other vice that was essential to sustaining me throughout the two months in Turkey? It was the television. Yep, I felt like a complete and total couch potato. Except I was lying in a hospital bed getting more chemotherapy drugs than any one person should have to endure. You may recall that I said the only two channels on Turkish television in English were news channels, but it can get really old (not to mention depressing as hell) listening to news. So we give thanks today for iTunes, a universal DVD player, a laptop, and that the BBC took a break from the news and offered American television shows for two hours a night.

Liz and I became hooked on Dexter, Burn Notice, Rizzoli and Isles, Modern Family, and The Middle. iTunes allowed us to stay current with our all-time favorite, NCIS, and buy seasons of other shows we got hooked on. I got through the roughest of days knowing we had a plethora of such distractions at our fingertips. After all, it was Turkey where I discovered MasterChef and those amazing contestants who changed my life in ways I never could have imagined.

Liz was also my connection to maintaining a healthy mind throughout the entire process. Every day, three times a day, I was required to walk the transplant ward for at least twenty minutes. While this was the only time I could really leave my isolation chamber, trust me when I tell you that the energy wasn't always there to do it. Liz kept me going. We used that time to talk about our dreams, and we started making lists of our plans. Liz would ask me specifically what else I wanted to put on my bucket list since we had done the top three before we knew I would actually get my transplant.

This walking therapy, as I called it, also helped me to change my thinking from having a bucket list to having a life list. All my life, I had a bucket list, like many of us do, that list of things we really want to do or see before we die.

For me it made perfect sense, I was spending a good portion of my days waiting to die. But now? Now I had hope. With the realization that I was getting a new life, or a do-over, we thought it was best to really embrace the idea of a new, fresh positive.

Not that my bucket list was negative in any way, shape, or form. It consisted of all kinds of once-in-a-lifetime goals and dreams. It was just that everything on my bucket list were things I wanted to do before I died. Now—now I was going to live. Or at least live a life where my focus could be on things that I always wanted to do but never really thought I would have time to do. Or things that would seem mundane, or just simple, to those folks who might not ever have experienced a do-over or second chance in life like I was getting. This was a chance for me to re-channel my views on what's important.

When Liz and I first met, my bucket list was kind of short. Not because I didn't dream or have goals, but I had spent a lot of time trying to check things off that list

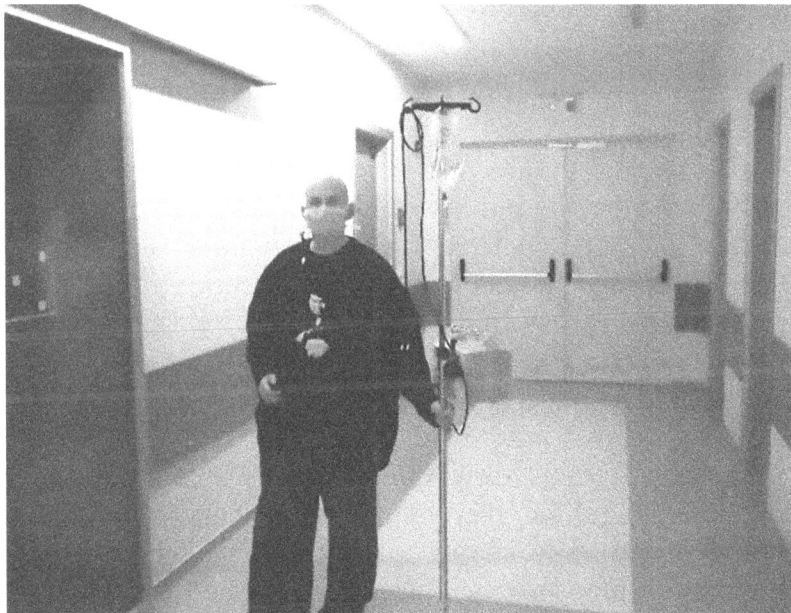

Walking and thinking; planning a life list

so that only three remained. Number three was to go to Disneyland one last time. I would have preferred one more Christmas visit to Disney World, but I didn't think I had that kind of energy left.

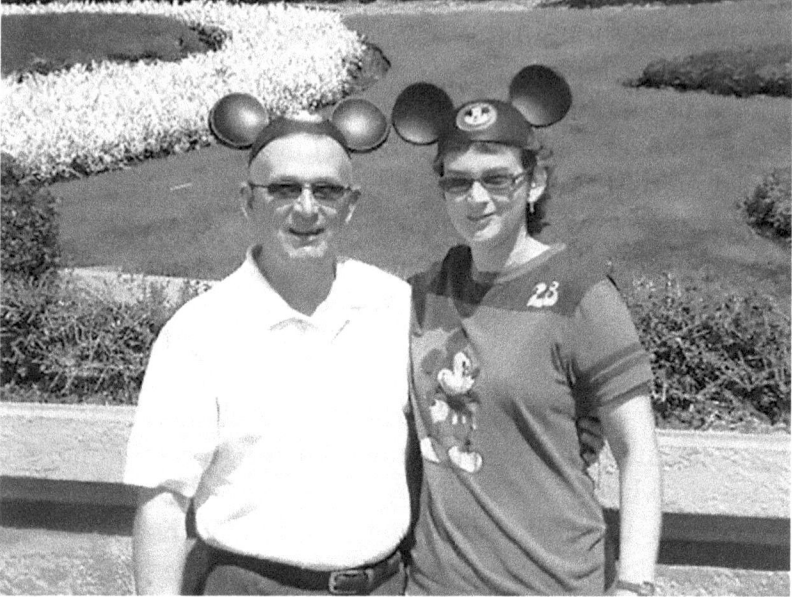

Maybe it's all those good memories of Cristy and her Dad, pre-transplant at Disney World

Why Disney World or Disneyland? I'm not altogether sure what it is about those parks that appeals to me so. Maybe it's the action, the colors, the pulse of life, the innocence, and the pure joy that characterizes everything about those parks and everyone who visits or works there. Second on the list was to finally get tenure at UH. And number one on my bucket list—something that had not changed since I was in tenth grade World History—was to go to Vienna, Austria. Why Vienna? I'm not entirely sure about that either, but it held an enchantment for me that I can't explain. I really just wanted to see Vienna.

For me and Liz traveling to Disneyland and Vienna was a way to build lasting memories for us as a couple, but for me, alone, getting tenure was that final professional goal I wanted next to my name so no one could ever call me a quitter. As it would happen, we accomplished all three things before it was time to leave for Turkey. It wasn't always easy, but it was worth the effort.

As the saying goes, "Out with the old and in with the new." Since my bucket list had been completed and I was given a new start, my list should also have a new beginning. So the life list was born in the halls of the transplant ward at Anadolu Medical Center half a world away from home.

My life list began as a list of things to look forward to as soon as we got home. Things that we were missing while in Turkey. Funny, though. My life list is not exactly a list. For now, my life list is mostly in my head, but it is kind of like my T-Charts. I tend to categorize my list into those that are in the now and those that are a bit more long term. For example, one of my greatest joys now is the taste of food. Something happened to my taste buds during the transplant and now food tastes so vibrant and real. As a result, my life list always has new places to eat or new foods to try. Of course, these are things that change frequently, and that, my friends, has its benefits. Each time I get to

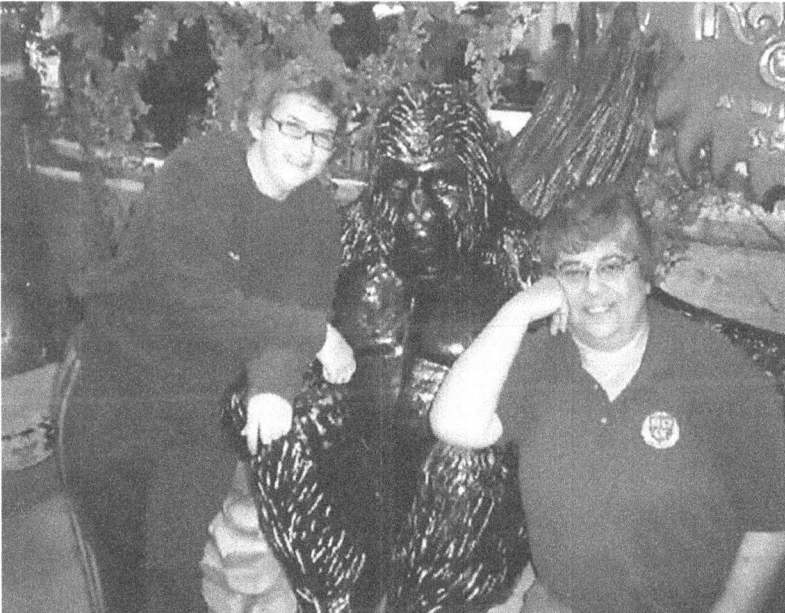

Cristy and Liz with a friend at the Rainforest Cafe, Disneyland

check one of those places or a type of food off my list, I feel a sense of accomplishment. But even bigger than that, they remind me, shall we say, to stop and smell the roses. And they remind me that I am not racing against the clock of fate; I can take my time and take detours any time I want. There is no deadline.

On the long-term side, the first thing that went on my list was to write a book. So I guess as I get close to checking that off, I am reminded of the things I am passionate about and the things that matter in this, my new life. It is my greatest hope that by opening the spy glass into my personal journey, you will find something that encourages you to stop and find what it is that can sustain you during your life's journey.

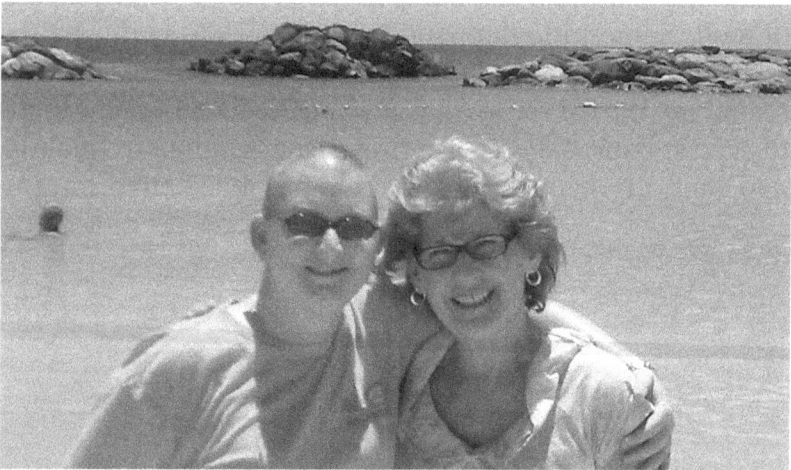

Cristy and her mother, post-transplant in Hawaii. How do you say "Thank You"?

CHAPTER 7—AFTERWORD

It is no exaggeration when I say I would not be here today writing this book if I had not taken charge of my own medical care and become my own patient advocate.

It's true that along the way there were others, professional advocates whose services were vital, but I am convinced that my own efforts were instrumental in getting the medical care I needed to save my own life. Each of the autoimmune diseases I had was potentially fatal.

There is no cure for scleroderma, and in most patients, the disease slowly gets worse. If the symptoms only affect the skin, the prognosis is better, but it can damage the heart, kidney, lungs, or GI tract, which may cause death.

Hollywood celebrities Bob Saget and Jason Alexander have become advocates for scleroderma research. Saget's sister died from the disease, as did Alexander's mother, and his sister suffered from scleroderma for thirteen years before she was properly diagnosed. "My doctor told me that there was nothing wrong with me that a new boyfriend and a yoga class wouldn't cure," she said.[1]

I can identify with that kind of cavalier attitude.

Ankylosing spondylitis is an inflammatory disease of the skeletal system. It affects the entire body, but the spine, which can fuse together, and the hips are particularly affected. Other organs, such as the heart, lungs, kidneys, colon, and eyes can be affected. In cases where circulatory disease is present, death is more likely.[2]

And speaking of circulatory disease, vasculitis refers to a group of rare diseases that have in common

1   http://nihrecord.od.nih.gov/newsletters/06_25_2002/story05.htm
2   www.medscape.com/viewarticle/751105

inflammation of blood vessels. Symptoms can be mild to life threatening.[3]

Yes, any one of these diseases is potentially fatal, and in combination the odds of survival were stacked against me. I knew it was just a matter of time and that if I couldn't always get the answers I needed from my doctors, I had to take charge. That determination led to these five steps:

- **Step 1: Sensibility**—Listen to your body and learn how to interpret what it has to tell you so you can share this information with your doctors.

- **Step 2: Teamwork**—Build a team of medical practitioners and a family and friends support network that communicates well and works together for the same goals.

- **Step 3: Education**—Learn everything you can about the symptoms, disorders, diseases that you may be facing as well as the treatments available; become an expert on you.

- **Step 4: Patience and Perseverance**—Don't expect things to happen quickly, but don't give up; know when to push for more timely information and treatment.

- **Step 5: Sustainability**—This is all about you and what you need to take care of and protect your body, mind, and spirit. It involves deep thought and reflection to determine what you need in your life that will help you keep going day after day after day.

Early in this book, I said my transplant and my story are unique, but I suspect that dealing with multiple autoimmune diseases may not be all that unique, and that really scares me. I don't want you to struggle through a medical maze for over twenty years before figuring out that your own best patient advocate is yourself.

---

3   www.rheumatology.org/Practice/Clinical/Patients/Diseases_And_Conditions/Vasculitis

I hope this little book will not only *save* you time, but *give* you more time.

ABOUT THE AUTHORS

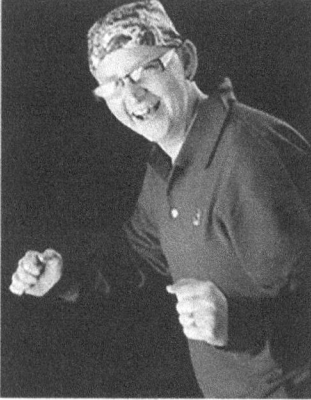

Cristy Kessler's message is one of hope. While living with incurable diseases and unbearable pain that would have crippled most of us, Cristy managed to achieve her dream of becoming a tenured university professor and also be the only tenure-line faculty member at the University of Hawaii to hold National Board Certification. Being told there was nothing more that could be done to keep her body from suffocating itself from scleroderma, ankylosing spondylitis, and vasculitis, Cristy was waiting to die. Fighting to live and remain teaching led Cristy on the journey to find her own cure; to be her own health care advocate. To hear her story is to hear a story of joy and faith.

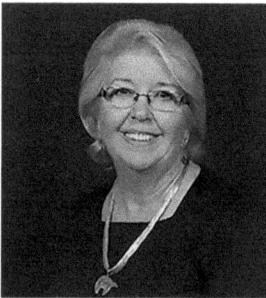

Sharon Miller, owner of Buckskin Books, is a freelance writer and editor, specializing in working directly with authors who wish to self-publish print and e-books. A former English teacher and close personal friend of Cristy Kessler, she volunteered and contributed hours of time and resources to raising money for Cristy's medical expenses. Working with Cristy on this book has been pure pleasure. It is a story worth telling many times over.

MEDICAL GLOSSARY

Adenocarcinoma

Definition: Adenocarcinoma is the second most common to 20 percent of all cervical cancers. Cervical adenocarcinoma arises within glands located in the endocervix. The most common subtype of cervical cancer, called squamous cell carcinoma, arises from the surface lining of the ectocervix, usually at the area where the ectocervix connects to the endocervix. If not successfully treated at an early stage, cervical cancer is capable of invading through the wall of the uterus into adjacent areas and sometimes can spread through the bloodstream or the lymphatic system to parts of the body away from the uterus.

Symptoms: Abnormal bleeding from the vagina, including bleeding between periods or spotting/bleeding after menopause. Extremely long, heavy, or frequent episodes of vaginal bleeding after age 40. Lower abdominal pain or pelvic cramping; thin white or clear vaginal discharge after menopause.

Treatment: Treatment involves surgery, radiation therapy, and chemotherapy. Removal of the uterus (hysterectomy) may be done in women with early stage 1 uterine cancer. Removal of the tubes and ovaries is usually recommended. Surgery combined with radiation therapy is often used to treat women with Stage 1 disease that has a high chance of returning, has spread to the lymph nodes, or is a Stage 2 or 3. It is also used to treat women with stage 2 disease. Chemotherapy or hormonal therapy may be considered in some cases, especially for those with

Stage 3 disease.
Source: www.nlm.nih.gov/medlineplus/ency/arti-
cle/000910.htm

*Ankylosing Spondylitis**

**An autoimmune disease for which stem cell
transplant has not been approved in the United
States.*

Definition: Ankylosing spondylitis is a type of arthritis of
the spine. It causes swelling between your vertebrae and
in the joints between your spine and pelvis. Ankylosing
spondylitis is an immune disease. Over time, it can fuse
your vertebrae together, limiting movement. Symptoms
can worsen or improve or stop altogether. The disease has
no cure, but medicines can relieve the pain, swelling and
other symptoms. Exercise can also help.
Symptoms: Symptoms usually start to appear in late
adolescence or early adulthood (ages 17-35); the symptoms can occur in children or much later. Typically, the
first symptoms of AS are frequent pain and stiffness in
the lower back and buttocks, which comes on gradually
over the course of a few weeks or months. At first, discomfort may only be felt on one side, or alternate sides.
The pain is usually dull and diffuse, rather than localized.
This pain and stiffness is usually worse in the mornings
and during the night, but may be improved by a warm
shower or light exercise. Also, in the early stages of AS,
there may be mild fever, loss of appetite and general
discomfort. It is important to note that back pain from
ankylosing spondylitis is inflammatory in nature and
not mechanical. The pain normally becomes chronic and
is felt on both sides, usually persisting for at least three
months. Over the course of months or years, the stiffness
and pain can spread up the spine and into the neck. Pain
and tenderness spreading to the ribs, shoulder blades,
hips, thighs and heels is possible as well. In a minority
of individuals, the pain does not start in the lower back,

but in a peripheral joint such as the hip, ankle, elbow, knee, heel or shoulder. This pain is commonly caused by enthesitis, which is the inflammation of the site where a ligament or tendon attaches to bone. Inflammation and pain in peripheral joints is more common in juveniles with AS. Advanced symptoms can be chronic, severe pain and stiffness in the back, spine and possibly peripheral joints, as well as lack of spinal mobility because of chronic inflammation and possible spinal fusion.

Treatment: A common treatment regimen involves medication, exercise and possibly physical therapy, good posture practices, and other treatment options such as applying heat/cold to help relax muscles and reduce joint pain. In severe cases of ankylosing spondylitis, surgery may also be an option.

Source: www.spondylitis.org/about/as_sym.aspx and www.spondylitis.org/about/treatment.aspx

Aseptic Necrosis

Definition: Aseptic necrosis is a condition that occurs when bone tissue dies because of too little blood supply. The bone eventually collapses after tiny breaks occur. In most cases, the condition affects the thighbone (femur) in the hip area, but it can affect other bones in the body. These areas include the wrist, knee, and shoulder. It worsens with time. The condition is also called osteonecrosis, avascular necrosis, or ischemic bone necrosis. Can be caused by long-term use of steroids or chemotherapy.

Symptoms: The condition may cause no symptoms; however, some people have pain or a loss of motion in the affected joint. In the hip, there may be groin pain that spreads down the thigh to the knee. In the wrist, the condition may cause wrist pain and weakness in the fingers. In the shoulder, it can result in pain and stiffness in the upper arm. In the knee, the condition can cause pain in the lower end of the thighbone.

Treatment: Reduced weight bearing—If the condition is diagnosed early, reduced weight bearing can be helpful in

removing weight from the affected joint. This may involve the use of crutches or the limitation of certain activities. Core decompression—Core decompression is a surgery in which the inner layer of bone is removed. This surgery is most effective for people in the earliest stages of the disease. Osteotomy—This surgery reshapes the bone in order to lessen stress on the area affected. The surgery is most effective for patients with advanced forms of the disease and when avascular necrosis affects a large area of bone. Bone graft—In this surgery, healthy bone is transplanted from one part of the patient to the area affected by avascular necrosis. This procedure is complex and its effectiveness has not yet been proven. Arthroplasty/total joint replacement—This treatment is used in late-stage avascular necrosis and when the joint is destroyed. The diseased joint is replaced with artificial parts.
Source: http://my.clevelandclinic.org/orthopaedics-rheumatology/diseases-conditions/hic-avascular-necrosis.aspx

Ativan

Ativan (lorazepam) is used to affect chemicals in the brain that may become unbalanced and cause anxiety. Ativan is used to treat anxiety disorders. Serious side effects: confusion, depressed mood, thoughts of suicide or hurting yourself, hyperactivity, agitation, hostility, hallucinations, or feeling light-headed, fainting. Less serious Ativan side effects: drowsiness, dizziness, tiredness, blurred vision, sleep problems (insomnia), muscle weakness, lack of balance or coordination, amnesia or forgetfulness, trouble concentrating, nausea, vomiting, constipation; appetite changes, or skin rash. **Source:** www.drugs.com

ATG

Anti-Thymocyte Globulin ATG is a special antibody that is used to treat aplastic anemia and graft-versus-host disease in patients having a stem cell transplant. It is given intravenously (IV). Serious allergic reactions including anaphylaxis can occur. **Source:** www.upmc.com/pa-tients-visitors/education/cancer-chemo/pages/anti-thy-mocyte-globulin.aspx

Bactrim

Bactrim contains a combination of sulfamethoxazole and trimethoprim, which are both antibiotics that treat different types of infection caused by bacteria. Side effects are too numerous to list here. **Source:** www.drugs.com

Chiari Malformation

Definition: Chiari malformations (CMs) are structural defects in the cerebellum, the part of the brain that controls balance. Normally the cerebellum and parts of the brain stem sit in an indented space at the lower rear of the skull, above the foramen magnum (a funnel-like opening to the spinal canal). When part of the cerebellum is located below the foramen magnum, it is called a Chiari malformation. CMs may develop when the bony space is smaller than normal, causing the cerebellum and brain stem to be pushed downward into the foramen magnum and into the upper spinal canal. The resulting pressure on the cerebellum and brain stem may affect functions controlled by these areas and block the flow of cerebrospinal fluid (CSF)— the clear liquid that surrounds and cushions the brain and spinal cord—to and from the brain. CM has several different causes. It can be caused by structural defects in the brain and spinal cord that occur during fetal development, whether caused by genetic mutations or lack of proper vitamins or nutrients in the maternal diet. This is called primary or congenital CM. It can also be caused later in life if spinal fluid is drained excessively from the lumbar or thoracic areas of the spine either due to injury, exposure to harmful substances, or infection. This is called acquired or secondary CM. The most common is Type I, which may not cause symptoms and is often found by accident during an examination for another condition. Type II is usually accompanied by a myelomeningocele-a form of spina bifida that occurs when the spinal canal and backbone do not close before birth, causing the spinal cord to protrude through an opening in the back. This can cause partial or complete paralysis below the spinal opening. Type III is the most serious form of CM, and causes severe neurological defects. Other conditions sometimes associated with CM include hydrocephalus, syringomyelia, and spinal curvature.

Symptoms: Individuals with CM may complain of neck pain, balance problems, muscle weakness, numbness or other abnormal feelings in the arms or legs, dizziness, vision problems, difficulty swallowing, ringing or buzzing in the ears, hearing loss, vomiting, insomnia, depression, or headache made worse by coughing or straining. Hand coordination and fine motor skills may be affected. Symptoms may change for some individuals, depending on the buildup of CSF and resulting pressure on the tissues and nerves. Persons with a Type I CM may not have symptoms. Adolescents and adults who have CM but no symptoms initially may, later in life, develop signs of the disorder. Infants may have symptoms from any type of CM and may have difficulty swallowing, irritability when being fed, excessive drooling, a weak cry, gagging or vomiting, arm weakness, a stiff neck, breathing problems, developmental delays, and an inability to gain weight. Some CMs are asymptomatic and do not interfere with a person's activities of daily living. In other cases, medications may ease certain symptoms, such as pain.

Treatment: Surgery is the only treatment available to correct functional disturbances or halt the progression of damage to the central nervous system. Most individuals who have surgery see a reduction in their symptoms and/ or prolonged periods of relative stability. More than one surgery may be needed to treat the condition. Posterior fossa decompression surgery is performed on adults with CM to create more space for the cerebellum and to relieve pressure on the spinal column. Surgery involves making an incision at the back of the head and removing a small portion of the bottom of the skull (and sometimes part of the spinal column) to correct the irregular bony structure. The neurosurgeon may use a procedure called electrocautery to shrink the cerebellar tonsils. This surgical technique involves destroying tissue with high-frequency electrical currents.

Source: www.ninds.nih.gov/disorders/chiari/chiari.htm

Conization

Definition: A cone biopsy is an extensive form of a cervical biopsy. It is called a cone biopsy because a cone-shaped wedge of tissue is removed from the cervix and examined under a microscope. A cone biopsy removes abnormal tissue that is high in the cervical canal. A small amount of normal tissue around the cone-shaped wedge of abnormal tissue is also removed so that a margin free of abnormal cells is left in the cervix.

Source: www.webmd.com/cancer/cervical-cancer/cone-biopsy-conization-for-abnormal-cervical-cell-changes

CREST Syndrome

Definition: This is a term applied to the symptoms of multiple autoimmune disorders.

Symptoms: The symptoms involved in CREST syndrome are associated with the generalized form of the disease systemic sclerosis (scleroderma). CREST is an acronym for the clinical features that are seen in a patient with this disease. The "C" stands for calcinosis, where calcium deposits form under the skin on the fingers or other areas of the body. The "R", stands for Raynaud's phenomenon, a spasm of blood vessels in the fingers or toes in response to cold or stress. The "E" represents esophageal dysmotility, which can cause difficulty in swallowing. The "S" is for sclerodactyly, tightening of the skin causing the fingers to bend. Finally, the letter "T" is for telangiectasia, dilated vessels on the skin of the fingers, face, or inside of the mouth.

Treatment: See treatment for the named autoimmune disorders.

Source: www.nlm.nih.gov/medlineplus/ency/imagepages/19507.htm

Cytoxan

Cytoxan (Cytoxin) is an antineoplastic medicine. It works by stopping or slowing the growth of malignant cells. Cytoxan (Cytoxin) may be used alone but is often given with other anticancer medications. Side effect include: appetite loss; absence of menstrual periods; color change in skin; diarrhea; general unwell feeling; hair loss; nausea; skin rash; stomach discomfort or pain; texture change in nails; vomiting; weakness. **Source:** www.drugs.com

Engraftment/Graft-versus-Host Disease

Definition: Graft-versus-host disease (GVHD) is a complication that can occur after a stem cell or bone marrow transplant in which the newly transplanted donor cells attack the transplant recipient's body. GVHD does not occur when someone receives his or her own cells during a transplant (called an autologous transplant). Engraftment is when the body accepts the stem cells.

Source: www.nlm.nih.gov/medlineplus/ency/article/001309.htm

Esophageal Dysmotility Disorder

Definition: The esophagus is a muscular tube that extends from the neck to the abdomen and connects the back of the throat to the stomach. When a person swallows, the coordinated muscular contractions of the esophagus propel the food or fluid from the throat to the stomach. If the muscular contractions become discoordinated or weak, interfering with movement of food down the

esophagus, this condition is known as a motility disorder.
Symptoms: Motility disorders cause difficulty in swallowing, regurgitation of food, and, in some people, a spasm-type pain.
Treatment: Two types of treatment are performed under sedation using endoscopic guidance. One, known as pneumatic dilation, involves placing a balloon in the swallowing passage at the level of the valve between the esophagus and stomach. This balloon is forcefully expanded, tearing the muscles of the valve so that the valve no longer obstructs passage of food from the esophagus into the stomach. This has a 75% chance of relieving symptoms for a period of years, but has a 3% risk of rupturing the esophagus. If esophageal rupture occurs, then emergency surgery is necessary to repair the rupture and then treat the achalasia surgically. The other type of treatment that is performed under endoscopic guidance is botulinum toxin, or Botox, injection. This toxin paralyzes the muscles of the valve between the esophagus and stomach, permitting food to pass from the esophagus into the stomach. Over 60% of people who have this therapy get substantial relief of symptoms for at least one year.
Source: www.sts.org/patient-information/esophageal-surgery/achalasia-and-esophageal-motility-disorders

Faces Pain Scale

Faces Pain Scale-Revised is from the International Association for the Study of Pain which allows patients to rate their pain on a scale of 1-10 based on drawings depicting facial expressions.
Source: www.iasp-pain.org/Content/NavigationMenu/GeneralResourceLinks/FacesPainScaleRevised/default.htm

HLA B27

Definition: HLA-B27 is a blood test to look for a protein

that is found on the surface of white blood cells. The protein is called human leukocyte antigen B27 (HLA-B27). Human leukocyte antigens (HLAs) are proteins that help the body's immune system tell the difference between its own cells and foreign, harmful substances.
Source: www.nlm.nih.gov/medlineplus/ency/article/003551.htm

Meckel's Diverticulum

Definition: MD is a pouch on the wall of the lower part of the intestine that is present at birth (congenital). The diverticulum may contain tissue that is the same as tissue of the stomach or pancreas. A Meckel's diverticulum is tissue left over from when the baby's digestive tract was forming before birth. A small number of people have a Meckel's diverticulum, but only a few develop symptoms.
Symptoms: Pain in the abdome that can be mild or severe; blood in the stool. Symptoms often occur during the first few years of life, but they may not start until adulthood.
Treatment: The segment of small intestine that contains the diverticulum is surgically removed. The ends of the intestine are sewn back together. Iron replacement is recommended to correct anemia. If bleeding has been severe, a blood transfusion may be necessary.
Source: www.nlm.nih.gov/medlineplus/ency/article/000234.htm

Methotrexate

MTX works by dampening the inflammatory process associated with active vasculitis. The aim of using MTX is to push the disease into remission (inactivity) as soon as possible, before the inflammation causes permanent organ damage. MTX is a serious medicine used to treat vasculitis. Without it, many forms of vasculitis would cause longer courses of illness and greater damage. Side Effects: nausea, mouth ulcers, pneumonitis (inflammation of the lungs), liver problems, anemia, Thrombocytopenia (low platelets), Leukopenia (low white blood cell count), increased risk of developing lymphoma (a type of cancer) **Source:** www.hopkinsvasculitis.org/vasculitis-treatments/methotrexate-mtx/

Morphine

An opioid pain medication, sometimes called a narcotic. Morphine is used to treat moderate to severe pain. Extended-release morphine is for use when around-the-clock pain relief is needed. Side effects are too numerous to list here. **Source:** www.drugs.com

Neupogen

Neupogen - also known as Filgrastim (rbe) - is a copy of a substance normally present in your body, called Granulocyte Colony Stimulating Factor or G-CSF. Using gene technology, Neupogen is produced in a specific type of bacteria, called E. coli. G-CSF is produced in the bone marrow and assists in the production of neutrophils, which are a type of white blood cell. Neutrophils help the body fight infections by surrounding and destroying the bacteria that cause them. G-CSF also helps neutrophils to do this work better. Neupogen is typically used to increase this number before stem cell collection. You may also receive Neupogen after a bone marrow or stem cell transplant, to help speed up your recovery. Side effects: Like other medicines, Neupogen may have unwanted side effects. Some side effects may be serious and need medical attention. Other side effects are minor and are likely to be temporary. **Source:** www.news-medical.net/drugs/Neupogen.aspx

Prednisone

Prednisone is a corticosteroid. It prevents the release of substances in the body that cause inflammation. It also suppresses the immune system. Prednisone is used as an anti-inflammatory or an immunosuppressant medication. Prednisone treats many different conditions such as allergic disorders, skin conditions, ulcerative colitis, arthritis, lupus, psoriasis, or breathing disorders. Side effects: hives; serious difficult breathing; swelling of your face, lips, tongue, or throat normal sleep problems (insomnia), mood changes; increased appetite, gradual weight gain; acne, increased sweating, dry skin, thinning skin, bruising or discoloration; slow wound healing; headache, dizziness, spinning sensation; nausea, stomach pain, bloating; or changes in the shape or location of body fat (especially in your arms, legs, face, neck, breasts, and waist). **Source:** www.drugs.com

Prilosec *OTC*

Omeprazole is in a group of drugs called proton pump inhibitors. It decreases the amount of acid produced in the stomach and is used to treat symptoms of gastroesophageal reflux disease (GERD) and other conditions caused by excess stomach acid. Omeprazole is generally well tolerated. **Source:** www.drugs.com

Raynaud's Syndrome (Phenomenon)

Definition: Raynaud's phenomenon is a condition in which cold temperatures or strong emotions cause blood vessel spasms that block blood flow to the fingers, toes, ears, and nose. Raynaud's phenomenon can be associated with other conditions. This is called secondary Raynaud's phenomenon. Most people with the condition are over age 30. Common causes are: arthritis and autoimmune conditions, such as scleroderma, Sjogren syndrome, rheumatoid arthritis, and systemic lupus erythematosus. **Source:** www.nlm.nih.gov/medlineplus/ency/article/000412.htm

Rituxan

Rituxan (Rituxin) is a monoclonal antibody. It interferes

with the growth and spread of certain types of white blood cells (B cells) in the body. This helps to decrease pain, swelling, and inflammation in certain patients with rheumatoid arthritis. It is used alone or in combination with other medicines. It is also used in combination with methotrexate to treat rheumatoid arthritis. Rituxan (Rituxin) can cause serious side effects, some of which can be life threatening, including: Progressive Multifocal Leukoencephalopathy (PML), infusion reactions, Tumor Lysis Syndrome (TLS), and severe skin reactions. Other serious and life-threatening side effects include: hepatitis B virus reactivation, heart problems, infections, and stomach and bowel problems. Common side effects during Rituxan infusions include: fever, headache, chills and shakes, nausea, itching, hives, cough, sneezing, and throat irritation or tightness. **Source:** www.drugs.com

*Scleroderma**

*An autoimmune disease for which stem cell transplant has not been approved in the United States.

Definition: Scleroderma means hard skin. It is a group of diseases that cause abnormal growth of connective tissue. Connective tissue is the material inside your body that gives your tissues their shape and helps keep them strong. In scleroderma, the tissue gets hard or thick. It can cause swelling or pain in your muscles and joints. No one knows what causes scleroderma. It is more common in women. It can be mild or severe. Doctors diagnose scleroderma using your medical history, a physical exam, lab tests, and a skin biopsy. There is no cure, but various treatments can control symptoms and complications.
Symptoms: Symptoms of scleroderma include calcium deposits in connective tissues, Raynaud's phenomenon, (a narrowing of blood vessels in the hands or feet), swelling of the esophagus, thick, tight skin on your fingers, red spots on your hands and face.

Treatment: There are a number of treatments available to address the various conditions associated with scleroderma. None of these is a cure – they are designed to treat symptoms of the disease. A number of classes of drugs are currently approved, either in the US or Europe, to treat each condition. All medications have side effects that vary in severity.

Source: www.nlm.nih.gov/medlineplus/scleroderma. html#cat3

Stem Cell Transplant, Autologous

Definition: Stem cells are collected from the patients themselves, harvested, frozen and stored, then given back to the patient after intensive therapy. An autologous stem cell transplant is different from an allogeneic stem cell transplant, which uses stem cells from a matching donor. Source:www.cancercenter.com/treatments/autologous-stem-cell-transplant/

Stem Cell Transplant, Peripheral Blood

Definition: A stem cell (blood or marrow) transplant is the infusion, or injection, of healthy stem cells into your body to replace damaged or diseased stem cells. A stem cell transplant may be necessary if your bone marrow stops working and doesn't produce enough healthy stem cells. A stem cell transplant also may be performed if high-dose chemotherapy or radiation therapy is given in the treatment of blood disorders such as leukemia, lymphoma, or multiple myeloma. A stem cell transplant can help your body make enough healthy white blood cells, red blood cells or platelets, and reduce your risk of life-threatening infections, anemia and bleeding. Although the procedure to replenish your body's supply of healthy blood-forming cells is generally called a stem cell transplant, it's also known as a bone marrow transplant, peripheral blood stem cell transplant or an umbilical cord blood transplant, depending on the source of the stem

cells. Stem cell transplants can use cells from your own body (autologous stem cell transplant), from a donor (allogeneic stem cell transplant) or from an identical twin (syngeneic transplant).
Source: www.mayoclinic.com/health/stem-cell-transplant/MY00089

Syringomyelia

Definition: Syringomyelia is a rare disorder that causes a cyst to form in your spinal cord. This cyst, called a syrinx, gets bigger and longer over time, destroying part of the spinal cord. It usually results from a skull abnormality called a Chiari I malformation. A tumor, meningitis or physical trauma can also cause it.

Symptoms: Damage to the spinal cord from the syrinx can cause symptoms such as pain and weakness in the back, shoulders, arms or legs, headaches, inability to feel hot or cold. Symptoms vary according to the size and location of the syrinx. They often begin in early adulthood.

Treatment: Surgery is the main treatment. Some people also need to have the syrinx drained. Medicines can help ease pain. In some cases, there are no symptoms, so you may not need treatment.
Source: www.nlm.nih.gov/medlineplus/syringomyelia.html

Telangiectasia

Definition: Telangiectasias are small, widened blood vessels on the skin. They are usually meaningless, but may be associated with several diseases. Telangiectasias may develop anywhere within the body but can be easily seen in the skin, mucous membranes, and whites of the eyes. Usually, they do not cause symptoms. However, some telangiectasias bleed and cause significant problems. Telangiectasias may also occur in the brain and cause major problems from bleeding.
Source: www.nlm.nih.gov/medlineplus/ency/arti-

cle/003284.htm

Trigger Finger

Definition: also known as stenosing tenosynovitis (stuh-
NO-sing ten-o-sin-o-VIE-tis), one of your fingers or your
thumb gets stuck in a bent position and then straightens
with a snap — like a trigger being pulled and released. If
trigger finger is severe, your finger may become locked in
a bent position. Often painful, trigger finger is caused by a
narrowing of the sheath that surrounds the tendon in the
affected finger. Trigger finger more commonly occurs in
your dominant hand, and most often affects your thumb
or your middle or ring finger. More than one finger may
be affected at a time, and both hands might be involved.
Triggering is usually more pronounced in the morning,
while firmly grasping an object or when straightening
your finger.

Symptoms: Finger stiffness, particularly in the morning,
a popping or clicking sensation as you move your finger,
tenderness or a bump (nodule) at the base of the affected
finger, finger catching or locking in a bent position, which
suddenly pops straight, finger locked in a bent position,
which you are unable to straighten.

Treatment: Nonsteroidal anti-inflammatory drugs
(NSAIDs).Medications such as nonsteroidal anti-inflammatory drugs — ibuprofen (Advil, Motrin, others),
for example — may relieve the swelling constricting the
tendon sheath and trapping the tendon. These medications can also relieve the pain associated with trigger
finger. Steroids. An injection of a steroid medication, such
as a glucocorticoid, near or into the tendon sheath also
can be used to reduce inflammation of the sheath. This
treatment is most effective if given soon after signs and
symptoms begin. Injections can be repeated if necessary,
though repeated injections may not be as effective as the
initial injection. Steroid injections may not be as effective
in people with other medical conditions, such as rheumatoid arthritis or diabetes. Percutaneous trigger finger

release. In this procedure, which is performed with local anesthesia, doctors use a needle to release the locked finger. This procedure is most effective for the index, middle and ring fingers. Surgery. Though less common than other treatments, surgical release of the tendon may be necessary for troublesome locking that doesn't respond to other treatments.

Source: www.mayoclinic.com/health/trigger-finger/DS00155

*Vasculitis**

*An autoimmune disease for which stem cell transplant has not been approved in the United States.

Definition: Vasculitis is an inflammation of the blood vessels. It happens when the body's immune system attacks the blood vessel by mistake. It can happen because of an infection, a medicine, or another disease. The cause is often unknown. Vasculitis can affect arteries, veins, and capillaries. When a blood vessel becomes inflamed, it can narrow, making it more difficult for blood to get through, or it can close off completely so that blood can't get through at all. A blood vessel can stretch and weaken so much that it bulges. The bulge is called an aneurysm. If it bursts, it can cause dangerous bleeding inside the body.

Symptoms: Symptoms of vasculitis can vary, but usually include fever, swelling and a general sense of feeling ill. The main goal of treatment is to stop the inflammation. Steroids and other medicines to stop inflammation are often helpful.

Treatment: Common prescription medicines used to treat vasculitis include corticosteroids and cytotoxic medicines. Corticosteroids help reduce inflammation in your blood vessels. Examples of corticosteroids are prednisone, prednisolone, and methylprednisolone. Doctors may prescribe cytotoxic medicines if vasculitis is severe or if corticosteroids don't work well. Cytotoxic medicines

kill the cells that are causing the inflammation. Examples of these medicines are azathioprine, methotrexate, and cyclophosphamide. Sometimes both corticosteroids and cytotoxic medicines are prescribed. Certain types of vasculitis may require surgery to remove aneurysms that have formed as a result of the condition.
Source: http://www.nhlbi.nih.gov/health/health-topics/topics/vas/treatment.html

Vicodin

Vicodin contains a combination of acetaminophen and hydrocodone. Both medicines are pain killers. Hydrocodone is an opioid pain medication. An opioid is sometimes called a narcotic. Acetaminophen is a less potent pain reliever that increases the effects of hydrocodone. Vicodin is used to relieve moderate to severe pain. An allergic reaction to Vicodin, such as, hives; difficulty breathing; swelling of your face, lips, tongue, or throat is life threatening. In rare cases, acetaminophen may cause a severe skin reaction that can be fatal. This could occur even if you have taken acetaminophen in the past and had no reaction. **Source:** http://www.drugs.com

Zyrtec OTC

Zyrtec (cetirizine) is an antihistamine that reduces the effects of natural chemical histamine in the body. Histamine can produce symptoms of sneezing, itching, watery eyes, and runny nose. Zyrtec is used to treat cold or allergy symptoms such as sneezing, itching, watery eyes, or runny nose. Zyrtec is also used to treat itching and swelling caused by chronic uticaria (hives). An allergic reaction to Zyrtec includes hives; difficult breathing; swelling of your face, lips, tongue, or throat, which can be life threatening. Serious side effects: fast, pounding, or uneven heartbeat; weakness, tremors (uncontrolled shaking), or sleep problems (insomnia); severe restless feeling, hyperactivity; confusion; problems with vision; or urinating less than usual or not at all. Less serious side effects: diz-ziness, drowsiness; tired feeling; dry mouth; sore throat, cough; nausea, constipation; or headache. **Source:** www.drugs.com

TABLE OF ABBREVIATIONS

ANA	Antinuclear Antibodies
BFF	Best Friend Forever
CT/CAT Scan	Computed Tomography/Computer Axial Tomography
FDA	Food and Drug Administration
GI	Gastrointestinal
GP	General Practitioner
GYN	Gynecologist
MRI	Magnetic Resonance Imaging
OB/GYN	Obstetrician/Gynecologist
OTC	Over the counter (medications which do not need a prescription)
RN, BSN	Registered Nurse, Bachelor of Science in Nursing
SCT	Stem Cell Transplant
UH	University of Hawaii
UM	University of Maryland

RESOURCES

For Your Information

Anadolu Medical Center, in Affiliation with Johns Hopkins Medicine,
+90 262 678 52 03
www.anadolusaglik.org/en
Virtual Tour of AMC
www.anadolumedicalcenter.com/sanaltur/anadolusag-likgebze/english.html

WorldMed Assist
866-999-3848
www.worldmedassist.com

Celebrating Cristy's Survival

The Stem Cell Blog-Stem Cell Transplant Helps Hawaii Professor Live
www.thestemcellblog.com/2012/01/12/stem-cell-trans-plant-helps-Hawaii-professor-live

YouTube: (youtube.com/user/druhprof)
Celebrating One Year Post Transplant
www.youtube.com/watch?v=QQOsz-DB-N8
Cristy Kessler from Hawaii Won Her Battle by Stem Cell Transplantation
www.youtube.com/watch?v=GEk2AVKtotk

Cristy's Connections

Cristy's Website: www.cristykessler.com
Email: uhprof@gmail.com
Twitter: @DrUHProf
LinkedIn: www.linkedin.com/pub/dr-cristy-kessler/5a/866/7b8
Facebook: www.facebook.com/DrUHProf
One of Our Own Fund: www.oneofourownfund.org

To Arrange for Cristy to Speak at Your Function,
email her at uhprof@gmail.com

Medical Information

Blood and Marrow Transplant Information Network

BMT InfoNet
2310 Skokie Valley Road, Suite 104
Highland Park, IL 60035
888.597.7674
www.bmtinfonet.org/

Cancer Treatment Centers of America—Autologous Stem Cell Transplant

Phone: Oncology Information Specialist representatives are available 24 hours a day, every day. (800) 268-0786
Online Chat is available at the website
www.cancercenter.com/treatments/autologous-stem-cell-transplant/

Haematologica: The Hematology Journal—"Stem Cell Transplantation for Autoimmune Diseases"

via Giuseppe Belli 4, 27100 Pavia, Italy.
Phone: +39 0382 27129
E-mail: office@haematologica.org
www.haematologica.org/content/95/2/185.full

International Scleroderma Network
Scleroderma Hotline (English Only)
Toll Free U.S. 1-800-564-7099
Direct Line: 1-952-831-3091
International Scleroderma Network (ISN)
7455 France Ave So #266
Edina, MN 55435-4702
United States
www.sclero.org/

National Heart, Blood, Lung Institute-Vasculitis
Phone: 301-592-8573
For access to free Telecommunications Relay Services
(TRS), dial 7-1-1 on your telephone
NHLBI Health Information Center
P.O. Box 30105
Bethesda, MD 20824-0105
www.nhlbi.nih.gov/health/health-topics/topics/vas/
nhlbiinfo@nhlbi.nih.gov (Please include a valid return
e-mail address in the body of the message.)

National Institutes of Health—Autoimmune Diseases and the Promise of Stem Cell Based Therapies
9000 Rockville Pike, Bethesda, Maryland 20892
stemcells.nih.gov/info/scireport/pages/chapter6.aspx
Patients seeking information on participating in a clinical
trial at the NIH Clinical Center call 1-800-411-1222 or
e-mail http://clinicalstudies.info.nih.gov/contact-prpl.
html.

Spondylitis Association of America
PO Box 5872
Sherman Oaks, CA 91413
SAA Member Hotline - Toll Free (U.S. Only): 1-800-777-8189
Company Phone: 1-818-892-1616
www.spondylitis.org/about/as.aspx

US National Library of Medicine, National Institutes of Health—Autologous Stem Cell Transplantation in Autoimmune Disease

National Center for Biotechnology Information, U.S. National Library of Medicine 8600 Rockville Pike, Bethesda MD, 20894 USA

www.ncbi.nlm.nih.gov/pubmed/17961728

What Our Readers Say

Dr. Kessler provides a genuinely compelling and honestly scripted chronicle of her medical and personal journey. As a clinical psychologist who specializes in neuropsychology, I believe this story of perseverance, resilience and adaptability is a must-read for anyone interested in taking a dynamic role in their healing process, and improving their efficacy as a self-advocate. (Dr. Tracie Umaki)

Overall, VERY gripping, enlightening, and uplifting. (Ben Starr)

Healthcare providers can be incredibly frustrating and complex to deal with, especially when individuals are also having to cope with devastating illness, but Kessler offers common sense, practical tactics when dealing with doctors, allowing patients to feel in charge of their own health.... although the journey she describes would be somber for most, she is able to make light of her situation; her humor and good attitude seeps through the entire book; it is very encouraging... well done. (Maya Soetoro-Ng)

As I have been grappling with a progressive genetic disability, a condition that baffled more than one specialist before finally being pinned down, I can certainly relate to Kessler's frustration with the way things are typically handled. Each of her five steps will equip you with what is needed to successfully be your own advocate in this utmost area of importance, your own wellbeing.

One example is the use of the Internet for research, not only looking for the source of your illness, but also how to find help. How do I know this? The one that pinned down my disease correctly was me (later confirmed by a neurologist). As Kessler said in this book, build a team of practitioners and supporters, but also make good use of your own intelligence. (John C. Kennedy)

I loved this book. As a person with anxiety, and mental illness, I am constantly trying to be my own advocate. . . I think, the biggest takeway from the book is that no one person is ever alone. There's always someone who can benefit from your experiences if you're willing to share your story. Also, communication is key. Getting your various physicians to communicate with each other is half the battle of being your own health advocate. . . I also think the book goes beyond the general idea of "advocacy" being I-read-it-on-the-internet-so-it-must-be-true. . . and I think this book can help frustrated patients and doctors alike. (Heather on Goodreads)

5 STEPS Advocate

Inspired by Cristy's personal medical journey, our mission is to empower our clients and customers to speak and act for themselves and loved ones when needs arise. We are first to market a comprehensive and effective system for helping people to be prepared and empowered to act on their own behalf or on behalf of those they love.

Five STEPS Advocate

Teaches patients and their caretakers to embrace the 5 STEPS Principles and to recognize that Knowledge is Power;

- teaches patients and their caretakers how to open doors that have been shut by conventional health care systems;

- teaches patients and their caretakers how to move forward when fear and societal expectations promote inaction;

- creates an environment of hope for individuals with chronic or severe illness;

- empowers everyone to advocate for their own health care needs.

We do this by providing health care education through books, workshops, webinars, podcasts and consulting services to individuals and organizations concerned with illness, wellness and recovery.

The 5 S.T.E.P.S. are based on the following principles:

- We know what our bodies are telling us about our well being and we need the tools to communicate that clearly to our physicians.

- We, along with our doctors and our network of family and friends, collaborate and work as a team for the most effective medical outcomes.

- We do our own research regarding our medical issues and share our learning with team members who reciprocate with support and the sharing of knowledge.

- We are patient with our bodies, ourselves, and others; we persevere regardless of setbacks and obstacles we encounter.

- We recognize that our overall well being depends on sustaining not only the body, but also the mind and spirit.

Outreach includes:

- Keynote speeches and presentations by founder and author Dr. Cristy Kessler

- Author events, book signings and readings at bookstores

- In-person and digital workshops (offered in a variety of settings, such as, senior and assisted living facilities, hospitals, chronic illness networks, health care networks, and active retirement communities)

- Individual and private consultation

- Webinars, podcasts, video messaging

To arrange for Cristy to speak at your event contact

Deb Grisham Entertainment - Nashville TN
www.debgrishamentertainment.com
615-405-5380

MY HEALTH.
MY BODY.
MY VOICE.

www.5stepsadvocate.com

Visit our blog at
www.myhealthmybodymyvoice.com

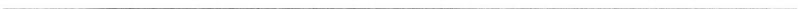